GENTLY DOW

GENTLY
DOWN *the*
STREAM

A PSYCHIATRIST'S LIFE

Jeffrey Hoffman

RADIUS BOOK GROUP

NEW YORK

Distributed by Radius Book Group
A Division of Diversion Publishing Corp.
443 Park Avenue South, Suite 1004
New York, NY 10016

www.RadiusBookGroup.com

First edition: 2018
Trade Paperback ISBN: 978-1-63576-561-8

Cover illustration by Augusto Argandona
Interior design and production by BookComp, Inc.

Printed in the United States of America
10 9 8 7 6 5 4 3 2 1

CONTENTS

CONTENTS

PREFACE

THIS MEMOIR IS INTENDED mainly as a gift to my family. It does not have the terrible adventures of my father or even the struggles experienced by my mother growing up as a Jewish girl in a small fishing town in northeastern Massachusetts. But it is my personal history, the story of what life was like growing up within a certain culture in the mid-twentieth century and what it was like to grow up in my family and to be educated and start a family and a practice on my own. I had loads of advice, some good, some not.

I hope that my children, grandchildren, and such friends and relatives who are interested in my story will enjoy it. And perhaps if premed or med students or people in the mental health professions come across it, it might reward their attention and interest as well. I hope so.

I've always been a reader, and while I have a proclivity for the comfort food of medical mysteries, legal thrillers, and spy novels, my nonfiction preferences in science and politics have affected my views a great deal, which will be apparent in the pages that follow.

Introduction

I AM NOT FAMOUS. I will not be remembered as a great scientist or humanitarian. Why write a memoir at all?

I have always enjoyed writing, and you are supposed to write about what you know best. What I know best is my family and my work.

Jake Hoffman, my paternal grandfather, deserted from Russian czar Nicholas II's army in about 1912. Jake left behind his teenage wife and baby son (my dad) and made his way to America with the intention of raising money so he could send for them and other members of the family. In about 1916, he finally had the money needed for his wife and son to travel. Unfortunately, World War I made it impossible for them to travel west, so Nana and my five-year-old dad headed east from their hometown in Ukraine, crossing Russia via the Trans-Siberian Railway to Vladivostok (longer than a round trip from Boston to Los Angeles). From there they made their way to Yokohama, Japan, where they waited six weeks for second-class steamship passage across the Pacific to Seattle. They finally joined Jake after traveling to Indiana, where he was working as a builder of passenger railway cars. Jake also paid for his younger brother, sister-in-law, two brothers-in-law, and father to make the journey. But the rest of his siblings and most of Nana's family chose to remain in Russia. As far as we know, they were all murdered by Hitler and the Nazis.

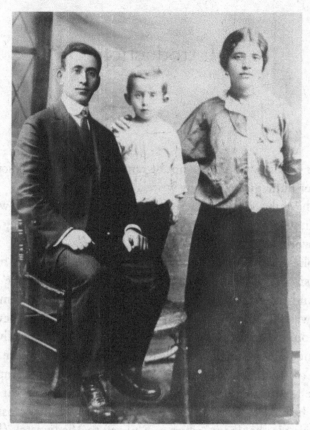

Zade, Nana, and Dad: New Immigrants

What an adventure for a little twenty-four-year-old Jewish lady, who only spoke Yiddish, and her five-year-old son! She must have been quite resourceful to survive that trip at all. How I would have loved to read about it! I would also have wanted to know more about my dad's experience in World War II, but I know that it was horrible, and writing about it would not have been helpful to him.

Mother grew up in Gloucester, Massachusetts, the youngest of four children—two sons and two daughters of George and

Ida Kline, who had immigrated to the United States from Bialystok in the early years of the twentieth century. Their eldest two children Robert and Miriam were born in the old country, and their son Irving was born in New York City. Mother was born in Gloucester in 1915.

George was a shoemaker by trade and learned that in Gloucester, where there were Jewish people, there was also work. He arrived there in 1907, having been preceded by about a dozen Jewish families. George's wife Ida was sickly and died many years before I was born, just before Mother graduated from Gloucester High School. I was named for Ida.

George was successful enough in the 1920s to send his eldest son Robert away to the Wharton School at the University of Pennsylvania. His older daughter, my aunt Miriam, married a few years out of high school to a Lowell, Massachusetts, boy named Max Gardner. Apparently George, like many, lost his business in the Great Depression, so going away to college was out of the question for Irving, who went to college and law school at nearby Boston University and struggled to make it as a lawyer in Gloucester, succeeding greatly only after World War II.

Mother was sent to Philadelphia to study oral hygiene at Temple University and live with her brother Bob, his wife Adele, and their little daughters Enid and Judy. Even in the best of times all of the Kline kids had to work to afford their education.

Family lore has it that when Bob and Adele quarreled, Bob would confide in his baby sister, my mom, who was a good listener, apparently earning the eternal enmity of her sister-in-law Adele. Nevertheless, my mother and dad married in May 1944 in Bob and Adele's house.

Bob became a very successful salesman. He was charming and outgoing. I remember Uncle Bob and Aunt Adele coming for visits to our home in Philly. He would chomp on his

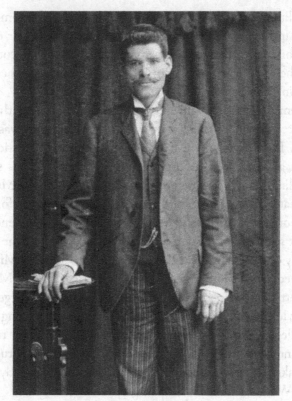

George Kline

ever-present cigar, and I would listen to lively discussions that were often political and heated but never angry. During the Kennedy-Nixon election of 1960, Mother once accused Bob of being a Republican, and Uncle Bob answered, "Your're goddamned right I'm a Republican." Aunt Adele was, at the time, a pretty middle-age woman, but I once saw a picture of her with Bob on a beach when they were in their twenties. She was drop-dead gorgeous, a natural beauty who looked a little like Ava Gardner.

While Mother never made any specific reference to any quarrels she and Adele may have had in the past, she often

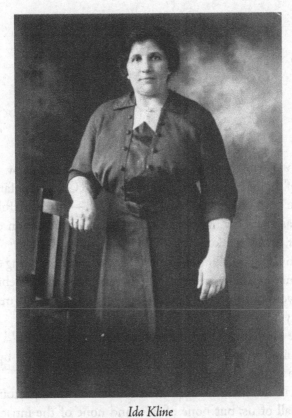

Ida Kline

warned me "Jeffrey, don't marry a beauty, you'll regret it," advice that I did not take and was wrong in my case.

Bob died suddenly of a heart attack at age fifty-nine in 1962. His wife and daughters were devastated, but after Bob's funeral we never saw any of them again for many years, until Judy came with her husband, an ear, nose, and throat doctor (ENT), and their three children from Cleveland, where they had settled, to Gloucester for one of our Fourth of July celebrations. Judy, also a Penn grad, became a psychiatric social worker, so we had a lot to talk about. She was cordial to Mother, but things were a little frosty between them.

February 10th

FANNY KAPLAN, Waldemar Hoven, Yuriy Poyarkov. Ever hear of them? Neither had I until I checked Google for famous people born on my birthday. Kaplan tried—unsuccessfully—to assassinate Lenin, Hoven was a Nazi concentration camp doctor, and Poyarkov was a Ukrainian volleyball player who was on Russia's Olympic team. Of course, I'm not being comprehensive. There are lots of other recognizable celebrities who were born on the same date I was and, for that matter, the day before and the day after.

The similarities and differences among them would look the same for any date you chose, utterly unaffected by the month or the day.

There are many forces in the universe that profoundly affect all of us, but none of us—and none of the intricacies of our personalities—were influenced by the position of the stars on the date of our birth, much less their anniversaries.

To me this is a primitive form of superstition, a holdover from the times (i.e., most of our existence as a species) when humans justifiably felt helpless dealing with forces of nature that could and did gratuitously kill us. And because we could neither comprehend nor control them, we made the understandable mistake of attributing intention to these forces or to planets, suns, and stars. If they were living gods, then maybe by prayer and supplication we could influence them to favor us. Unfortunately, most people think in a similar manner, calling it faith.

We are still battered by the forces of nature, but over the last few hundred years we have developed a better understanding of them, and that understanding has given us the capacity to have a little control over them as well.

Up until about thirty years ago, I would have described myself as agnostic.

Then, in no way intending to affect my religious beliefs, a friend recommended Richard Dawkins's book titled *The Blind Watchmaker*, which he wrote after his most famous book, *The Selfish Gene*. *The Blind Watchmaker* explains how complex biological structures (such as the eye) gradually come about in nature through the process of evolution (random mutations and natural selection) without any need for an external, conscious creator. Reading this thirty years ago essentially ended that kind of superstition for me.

But Dawkins and some of the other well-known professional atheists can be glib in pronouncing the wonders of science, and the process of discovery is spiritually satisfying. They mean this in the sense that the wonder and awe that they feel in the process of discovery sometimes brings about a feeling of transcendence that is similar to a profound religious experience. It's fine for the brilliant scientist who can grasp the mathematical reasoning behind scientific discovery and has the energy, curiosity, and ability to delve into it. Most people have neither the capacity nor the interest to experience science that way, and for them religious faith fills the need.

While not brilliant, I consider myself reasonably bright, and I enjoy reading books on scientific topics written for laymen. Frankly, I find that many of them take plenty of effort to follow and understand. I think that we are hardwired by evolution to experience faith and to not question authority, a good survival trait especially in childhood, when mindless obedience prevents the insertion of fingers into electric sockets.

I have enjoyed reading other popularizers of science such as Michio Kaku, Brian Greene, and Steven Hawking, physicists who write about cosmology and the Big Bang, string theory, quantum mechanics, the multiverse, and the elusiveness of a unified theory of the forces in the universe. I've also enjoyed reading Daniel Dennett, a philosopher of science who writes on the nature of consciousness, and Steven Pinker, a psychologist who writes about how the brain functions. Pinker, in particular, writes in a manner that's interesting to me, as I am a psychiatrist whose original training was greatly steeped in psychoanalytic theory, a body of observations and interpretations about the nature and treatment of mental illness that was never really subjected to scientific scrutiny.

When I was a senior medical student on my Adolescent Unit psychiatry elective, we were assigned a book that was neither a textbook nor a scientific paper. *The Abnormal Personality through Literature* was an anthology of short stories and excerpts from novels written by the greatest authors who ever lived. These were all descriptions or depictions of characters suffering from the range of mental illness, conveying their impact on the circumstances and people surrounding them. More compelling than any clinical description, these writings by authors including Chekhov, Hugo, Mann, Melville, Sartre, Fitzgerald, Poe, Dostoyevsky, Tolstoy, D. H. Lawrence, and many others enlivened the nature of the kinds of individuals who would one day be my patients. If I had to name one book that drew me to psychiatry, *The Abnormal Personality through Literature* was it.

There are those who divide science and theology into the study of what is versus what ought to be, but there are a number of authors, such as Sam Harris and Michael Shermer, who argue forcefully that ethics and right behavior can be deduced from our evolutionary past and how our brains function today.

Like many people, I consider myself spiritual in that I want to feel a connection between my little self and an indifferent universe, so vast compared to me.

Learning about the start of our universe over fourteen billion years ago as an unimaginably infinitesimal speck that expanded to amorphous clumps, which eventually became galaxies and stars, and about the formation of the heavy elements of Earth from exploding secondary stars, necessary for our kind of biological life to begin to exist, connects me to this process.

Reading about evolution and its hundreds of millions of years of fits and starts here on Earth gives me a better appreciation of how I came to be.

My little wink of self-awareness is amazing but sadly so brief and maybe even sadder because I know that I am on the lucky end of the spectrum of humans and perhaps all living creatures who have ever existed.

So, I try to enjoy the show and be good to the people who are important to me, even if they were not born on my birthday.

The following pages are my recollections of what happened after that day.

Lowell, Massachusetts

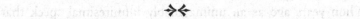

I WAS BORN IN LOWELL, Massachusetts, toward the end of World War II. Lowell was a working-class textile-factory town whose economy, though perhaps boosted by the war, was already in economic decline when I arrived.

Lowell was first settled in 1653 (then called Merrimack, the Indian name for its river). The town was incorporated as Lowell in 1826, named after an industrialist of the time. It became a city in 1836.

At the time of my birth, my mother was staying with her older sister Miriam and her brother-in-law Max, who was part owner of Depot Tire Service, a gasoline station and auto mechanic business. They had three sons, my cousins Donald, age sixteen; Howard, age nine; and David (little Doovy, whom my aunt particularly doted on), age seven. These cousins would all become an important part of my life.

My mother was staying with them while my dad was in a nearby army hospital recovering from wounds he had suffered as an infantryman in France in September 1944. My cousins felt a lifelong closeness to my mom based on those times. Family legend has it that Lowell suffered the worst snowstorm in its history at the time of my birth, and if it weren't for my cousin Donald digging her a path to the family car when she went into labor, I would have been born at their home at 492 Pine Street. This probably wouldn't have ended too well for me, since I was a breech baby.

Over the years, my mother, brother, and I spent several summers in Lowell when I was a child. On some weekends, my father made the drive from Philadelphia to visit us. Other weekends were spent on the beach in Gloucester, where we stayed with my bachelor uncle Irving in his tiny one-bedroom apartment. We happily gorged on eighty-five-cent lobster rolls sold at Bob's Clam Shack next door and visited with my grandfather, Grampy George, who was a shoemaker. Aside from owning Kline's Shoe Repair, he owned a couple of rental properties. He maintained his business and properties until well into his eighties.

I mentioned that Lowell was a factory town, but it had some nice residential areas. My aunt and uncle lived in a small white wooden house with a fairly large lawn in a leafy neighborhood, with a small local park nearby.

During the years before I turned twelve, my family lived in North Philadelphia in an urban neighborhood of pavement and brick that was rapidly turning dangerous. My parents, grandparents, and I all lived above the family business, Hoffman's Delicatessen.

To me, summer in Lowell was summer in the country. My aunt and uncle's house seemed gigantic, which I suppose it was compared to our home in Philly.

The Gardner family was always excited to see their cousins and nephews and always made my brother and me feel special and welcome. Aunt Miriam would make her famous chicken, and Uncle Max would boil corn. The dinners were raucous and delicious. There was a family dog, a Shetland sheepdog named Dike, who recognized me every summer, and we were absolutely inseparable.

Uncle Max swore at poor Dike constantly, unable to break him of his habit of chasing cars. I guess Max didn't realize that Shelties chase and herd by nature.

A number of boys close to my age lived in the neighborhood, and I don't remember exactly what we did except chasing frogs. Some of the boys went to camp during the day, but that didn't interest me, so I spent plenty of time just wandering around and playing with Dike. I didn't mind a bit.

One summer, my mom decided to take me downtown for social dancing lessons. I was embarrassed, and it resulted in plenty of gleeful teasing by my then teenage cousins. However, I did learn to cha-cha and jitterbug at the Lowell Dance Studio, the latter to numerous repetitions of "Daddy O" and "Dancing in My Socks," which have to be two of the worst jitterbug tunes of all time. I suppose the teacher must've thought that if the little twerp can learn to dance to this, he can dance to anything.

Our summers in Lowell ended in 1959 when Uncle Max, aged fifty-four, suffered a fatal heart attack. Soon thereafter, Aunt Miriam moved to Philadelphia to be close to my mother and her older son Donald, who had settled in the area.

I have many childhood memories of Lowell, only a few of which are recounted here, and they were happy.

Many years later when I settled in Massachusetts as an adult, I only went back to visit my "summer vacation home" once. It was tiny and painted garishly, and I felt no need to return. To me, Lowell is the town of my memories.

The Mansion

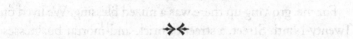

I WAS BORN IN LOWELL, where my mother lived for a few months during my father's wartime service. But until I was twelve, my family and I lived in a Philadelphia neighborhood called Strawberry Mansion, named after an actual mansion in Fairmount Park, one of the largest urban parks in the world and the western boundary of our North Philadelphia neighborhood. My parents, paternal grandparents, younger brother Ricky, and I all lived above the family business, Hoffman's Delicatessen. It was an old-fashioned deli with barrels of chips, pretzels, and pickles as well as yummy Tasty Cakes. The deli featured all kinds of spicy deli meats and Nana's homemade kosher cooking. I didn't like deli as a child, but I have more than made up for it since.

My grandparents doted on me and my brother, speaking to us mostly in Yiddish, a language I understood as a child but was not encouraged to speak, as it was rumored that my first words were pronounced like a greenhorn. In those days, proficiency in the language of your immigrant grandparents was not a high priority. This is a pity, as Yiddish is a beautiful, expressive tongue now spoken only in highly religious Jewish neighborhoods in a few large cities in the United States and Israel. My grandparents loved listening to old-fashioned Yiddish phonograph records, fabulous Jewish folk music called klezmer, which I didn't appreciate at the time but love to hear now.

My father clearly hated the business, but he was loyal to the owners, his parents, who expected him to be part of the family enterprise. My mother hated the neighborhood entirely. She wanted out badly, and when we finally moved in late 1956, I know that it was one of her happiest days.

For me, growing up there was a mixed blessing. We lived on Twenty-Ninth Street, a street of brick-and-mortar businesses. I grew up playing with the scions and heiresses of the owners of the local shoe store, candy store, clothing shop, awning shop, and tailor shop, so there were always kids to play with. I also acquired certain survival skills suitable to my modest stature. The mix of the neighborhood was perhaps 50 percent white, 40 percent black, and 10 percent Hispanic. Of the whites, about two-thirds were Jewish, but as the years went on the demographics changed in the usual direction. As a little kid, I was not acutely aware of specific racial or religious tensions. I think I was called a "sheenie" once, and I had no idea what it meant. I know that my non-Jewish friends sometimes made reference to their dads coming home drunk on Saturday night. They made light of it, but I'm sure they were often terrorized. My dad did not have to get drunk to have a similar effect on me.

In warm weather we played a form of stickball in the street called halfball, played with a cut-off broomstick for a bat and a hollow rubber ball called a pimple ball because its surface had pimply bumps. When the ball got old and lost its bounce, you cut it in half and played stickball with the hollow halfballs. A good halfball pitcher could put all kinds of spins and twirls on the halfball, and it took more than a little skill to connect the stick with the ball. The greatest hit was a roofer, which was when you hit a ball high enough to land on a roof. A roofer counted as five runs, and roofers lost us a lot of halfballs.

Once when I was walking home alone in the neighborhood, a neighborhood tough guy named Harry, a very large, menacing, Irish kid, approached me in a way that guaranteed there was a shakedown in store for me followed by a beating. So, I began a little prophylactic sniffing and sobbing.

"Sniff, sniff."

Harry asked, "What are you crying about, you little punk?"

"My pop, he bought me a pimple ball, and its on the roof, and, and my poppa's gonna beat me for losing it. Sniff, sniff."

I figured I had nothing to lose but my front teeth by over-estimating his stupidity. Maybe his father would beat him up for losing a pimple ball, and he'd be understanding. The kid actually felt sorry enough for me to go up on the roof and retrieve several halfballs and pimple balls. I know, I know. I was a cunning little bitch, but I did come home with my face intact and richer by a few rubber balls. Harry did not fare as well. He had a short life, most of which was spent in prison.

Boxing was quite popular then, and for men and boys watching the Friday night fights on TV was second in popularity only to watching the "Stinkin' Phillies," and its what I did regularly with my father and Zeda (Jake, my grandfather). Naturally, boxing was a popular playtime activity among boys in the Mansion, and though my family did its best to shelter me from the dangers of the neighborhood, engaging in bare-knuckle boxing matches was part of growing up there. These fights were generally friendly, although they were also used to settle disputes.

Once I got into it with a kid who was about my size for around twenty minutes. Apparently someone let Nana know what was going on, because there she was, shrieking loudly in Yiddish, breaking it up. Maybe I was embarrassed, maybe relieved, but I don't recall losing face. I guess most of the neighborhood kids had grandmothers.

My first neighborhood was a formative part of my life, despite my mother's concerted efforts to limit my exposure to it. Accordion lessons, swimming lessons, Hebrew school, and even elementary education all took place as far from the neighborhood as possible. At this point, a more properly grateful son might say "I'm glad she made me practice the accordion; it gave me a lifetime of pleasure." Sorry, no. It was torture, and

I haven't touched an accordion in sixty years. Religion and swimming haven't gone too well either.

My parents, however, were both avid bridge players. They never made an issue of it with me, but I have played duplicate bridge regularly through most of my life. Other interests I have, such as tennis, skiing, and to a lesser extent golf were acquired over the years.

I attended Hebrew school at Gratz, a great Philadelphia institution of Jewish learning with classes from kindergarten to graduate studies. So, of course Rick and I had to go—not just to bar mitzvah, my parents insisted, but through high school. One problem was that apart from Nana, my family had no interest in Jewish learning or taking religious practice seriously. We did not keep kosher or observe Shabbat, and aside from the high holidays (Rosh Hashana and Yom Kippur), we never went to synagogue. Once on Yom Kippur

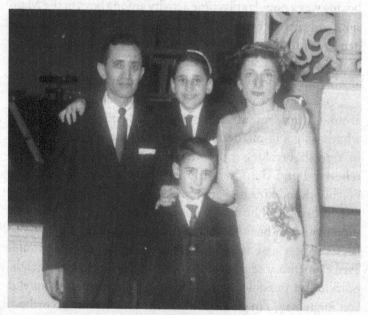

Jeff's Bar Mitzvah

(a day of fasting), my dad, who never fasted (headaches was his "medical" excuse), decided to call it a day from synagogue around lunchtime. He and I went to a nearby soda shop. I was about age ten and was hungry too.

I said, "Dad, I think I have a headache too, is it okay if I eat something?"

He answered, "Anything you want, Jeff."

"Even a BLT?" I ventured.

"Anything you want."

The BLT was delicious, and my family's view of religious observance was clarified forever.

Gratz was full of serious students, but I had no interest, never studied, and barely got by. However, it was the perfect place for my "bad boy" to come out. The teachers were mostly high school or college kids. One was Miss Klein, a pretty college girl with whom I may have been a little smitten. One afternoon I was wearing my Bermuda shorts under my long pants (I'd been in a public school play, where the shorts were part of the costume). In the middle of Miss Klein's class I stood up and removed my pants. The girls shrieked, the boys laughed, and Miss Klein immediately sent me to see Mrs. Elsie Chomsky, the very strict school principal. Like Charlie Brown in the Coasters' song, I innocently asked, "What'd I do wrong? It was hot in there." One of the kids later told me that Miss Klein told the class that they should feel bad for me because I was mentally ill. Later when I came home, my parents greeted me at the back of the deli. I don't remember what they said or did, but it couldn't have been good.

Mrs. Chomsky (the "ch" is pronounced gutturally, as in Hebrew) was a short, thin, wiry bundle of energy and a take-no-prisoners educator who ran the school with an iron fist. She was highly opinionated, a Labor Zionist by political conviction, and if you disagreed with her, you were wrong. People either venerated her or hated her, and you can guess where I stood. Her husband William was a brilliant Hebrew-language scholar who, among other things, was one of the pioneers in the development of modern Hebrew grammar. I remember him as a silent lurking presence who sometimes roamed the halls and classrooms of the school. Both were ardent Zionists. They had two sons, one who became a physician and the other, Noam, who in his early years was a pioneering linguistic genius and in later years has become the gadfly of American culture and an Israel-bashing ingrate. Ironic!

I was a great disappointment to Mrs. Chomsky, who thought that I was bright enough to go on to Gratz College and really learn something. Instead I went to the normal school, a kind of "Gratz College Lite" from where I graduated with a certificate qualifying me to teach Hebrew school to the second grade. I never used it.

We had little money to spare, so weekend entertainment generally involved visiting friends and family. My parents had loads of friends with kids close in age to Rick and me, so while the grownups talked we'd play, having lots of fun that didn't cost anything.

We also belonged to a cousins club, the "Menasha and Etta Factor Family Circle," named after Nana's parents. Every month we would go to someone's house and later a hired hall, where the men would play pinochle, the women would talk, and the kids played. Each June we had a cousin's club outing in Atlantic City, which was the highlight of the year.

After Fern and I married, I took her to a family circle meeting where my cousin Cookie, who was now married and living in Cherry Hill, New Jersey, was doing her part to carry on the family circle tradition. Unfortunately, my skinny Zeda, age eighty-one and standing all of 5'3", got into a pinochle brawl with a forty-something hothead who weighed in at well over two hundred pounds and was married to one of my cousins. The two were rolling on the floor before the fight was mercifully broken up and fortunately before someone got hurt. That was our last family circle.

One choice my parents made that worked out well was to send me out of the neighborhood to an elementary school, where I went from kindergarten onward. The local school, just around the corner, had a deservedly terrible reputation. There were no charter schools, and my parents were in no position to send me to a private school.

Mother found an alternative, the Thaddeus Stevens School, previously called the Old School of Practice because in the past it had been the school for training teachers in elementary education, and student teachers used to do their practice teaching there. I had to take a trolley and a subway to get there, but it was in general a good public school, open to children from anywhere in Philadelphia. It was racially mixed but was made up of youngsters whose parents wanted better for them. In second grade I got a well-deserved U (Unsatisfactory) in social habits for talking too much. I had a little crush on the teacher, Mrs. Perry.

In those days, nobody made a fuss about manhandling (boyhandling?) unruly pupils, and disseminating shaken-child syndrome was my third-grade teacher's preferred form of discipline. On my first day in her class, I wept out of sheer terror. She was really effective at it, but she also turned out to be an excellent teacher. She never shook me, as I was mostly too terrorized to say anything out of turn, let alone misbehave. And I got an O (Outstanding) in social habits.

The following year, I was out of school for over a month with rheumatic fever. I was hospitalized at the Children's Hospital of Philadelphia, and my doctor was a world-famous pediatrician of the time named Joseph Stokes, so I was probably sicker than I remember feeling. I was on antibiotics for about two years after that. My parents had told me that I had a sinus infection, and it was only years later when I discussed

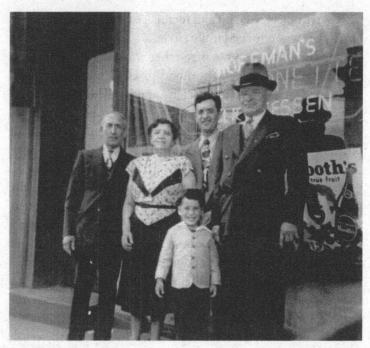

Nana, Zeda, Dad, Gramps, and Yours Truly in front of "the store"

what had happened with one of my professors in med school that we both concluded I'd probably had rheumatic fever (albeit a fairly mild case). Considering what nervous wrecks they were, I actually suspect that Dr. Stokes might have misled my parents as to my diagnosis. Doctors could probably get away with that back then. I was never hugged tighter or longer by a teacher as I was by my fourth-grade teacher, Mrs. Titus, on the day I returned to school.

Because there were so many students in the Philadelphia schools in the 1950s, graduations were staggered. And there were January and June graduates each year. Because of my birthday, I was a January grad. My mother felt that it would be an advantage for me to graduate in June, which would require me to skip the second half of the fifth grade. I'm no genius, but

I was a very good student, and I'm sure I could have managed to do sixth-grade work without the tutoring required by school regulations. But rules were rules, and so I qualified for the sixth grade after weeks of useless review of fifth-grade work.

The most prestigious organization available to fifth- and sixth-grade boys was membership in the safety patrol, and the most sublime post was "captain of the safeties." If you were on the safety patrol you were essentially a crossing guard, but somehow it was a very big deal to us. You got to wear a white belt and a shoulder strap with a silver badge pinned to it. I wasn't appointed in the first half of the fifth grade, and I skipped the second half. When I started the sixth grade the teacher didn't really know me, so in the first half of the year once again I wasn't appointed. Finally in the second term, I was a safety. I loved it and took it seriously, and I proudly wore my belt and my little silver badge. At the end of the term, the other boys assured me that if I weren't graduating, I would have been elected captain of the safeties for sure.

I wanted to be left back, but it was not to be. Eventually I'll get over it.

Lynnewood Road

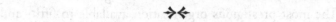

IN LATE 1956, our family finally moved out of the Mansion. Living there was getting to be a strain especially on Mother, whom I suspect may have resented my dad's devotion to a failing family business. The neighborhood was becoming less safe, and lots of our friends and neighbors had already moved to better parts of the city. One choice was Oxford Circle, a partly Jewish working-class neighborhood in the near northeastern part of Philly with affordable homes in the range of ten to twelve thousand dollars, mostly row houses. Mother was a bit of a snob and had her eye on the West Oak Lane/Mount Airy district of Philadelphia. Some of my parents' friends already lived there: the Litzes and the Muldowers. Max Litz was a milkman who had once rented from my grandparents, and Milt Muldower was an internist who was to be our family doctor for many years.

My father paid $13,300 for our semidetached house on Lynnewood Road. We were going upscale. To say that my parents were relieved is putting it mildly. No row house, no Oxford Circle for us! Our street was leafy, with young oaks and small lawns. Its inhabitants were mostly younger Jewish couples, many with very young children, thus providing my first major source of income, babysitting, at 50 cents per hour.

My new school was Morris E. Leeds Junior High, named for a trucking magnate. Leeds was a recently opened modern 1950s structure. When the teacher introduced short, skinny me to my homeroom, I suspect that the girls were disappointed and the boys were unimpressed. The class was all white, mostly Jewish with a smattering of other ethnic groups. The only thing integrated was academic ability, from fairly bright to pretty stupid.

At that time in Philadelphia, there was a well-known musical prodigy named Glenn Derringer, a dazzling accordionist and organist who appeared on local and national TV. I was vaguely aware that he had a sister who was almost as good an accordionist as he was and sometimes did duets with him on TV. When I started at Leeds I was suffering through accordion lessons, having no talent and less interest. Mother believed that if I practiced enough I'd get good, and besides, it would be a wonderful social asset. Coincidentally, I attended the accordion school where Glen Derringer had gotten his start.

A few days after I started at Leeds, our homeroom teacher decided to have a show-and-tell so we could "get to know each other better." Since I was the new kid, I was called on first. I had no idea what to say, but after a few forgettable remarks I mentioned that I played the accordion and took lessons at the same school that Glenn Derringer used to go to. I guess I thought that would impress them.

A few minutes after the show-and-tell, a pretty girl with bangs who was in my homeroom approached me. "Hi, I'm Brenda Derringer, Glenn's sister. Maybe we can play together sometime," she said. Talk about stepping in it. While my classmates were thinking "Oh, he takes lessons at Glenn's school. How nice!" all I could think of was how I could move back to the Mansion.

I told Brenda that I'd love to sometime, despite knowing that I'd sooner shoot myself.

There was a kid in my class named Eric who was teased and bullied somewhat. He was kind of aloof and a bit effeminate, and he was a poor athlete. I felt sorry for him, but I thought that his aloofness encouraged the teasing. Rick was to become a lifelong friend.

The second crush of my life was on Gloria, another girl in my homeroom. She had an adorable smile with which she flirted shamelessly. It didn't take very many smiles directed my way for me to become thoroughly smitten. But she had lots of boyfriends, and I kept my feelings to myself.

The teachers were mostly pedestrian and forgettable, but there was a shop teacher, Mr. Rysneczyk, who was notoriously intimidating. He was well over six feet tall and had a loud, angry voice. Once between classes we were as usual being unruly and noisy, and we were running in the hall. Mr. Rysneczyk came out into the hall, yelling in his booming voice "Slow down and walk!" My back was to him, and I was startled and started to laugh, and then heard Mr. R. shout, "Hey, Smiley, come here." There were so many other kids there that I didn't think he could have been referring to me, so I kept walking. Next thing I knew, I felt a large hand gripping my neck and slamming my back against the corridor wall. I was more stunned than hurt, but when I told my parents the reason for my detention and the events leading up to it, my father, who had a quick temper anyway, was enraged. He was the only one who had the right to maul his son.

The next morning, Dad stormed into Leeds fully intending to beat up Mr. R. (who stood a head taller and outweighed him by about forty pounds). Fortunately, Mother and I convinced him to stop by the counselors' office first. Mr. Shapiro, who was a social acquaintance of my parents, explained to Dad that Mr. R. had emotional problems (don't they all?) and that I could return to school without a bad mark on my record. Mr. R., of course, never changed, but I kept away from him.

My most (only) triumphant moment at Leeds came in the eighth grade when I was in the school play, a non-Pulitzer Prize–winning production of *Mr. Fixit*. I played the wise-cracking little brother and had most of the funny lines.

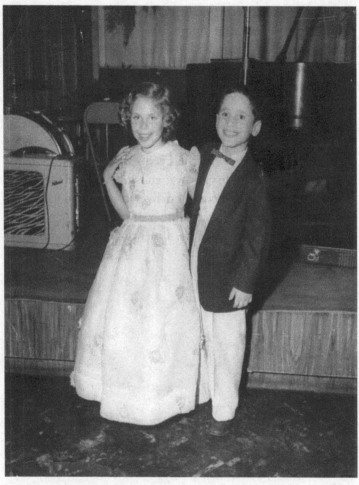

First Love Alice

    I mentioned that Gloria was my second crush. My first was a girl named Alice. I had first met Alice when I was eight years old when she was the flower girl at the Litzes' older daughter Etta's wedding. I guess that Alice was taken with me too, and we had a picture of us taken together, my arm around her, my face beaming. I called her the day after the wedding and had absolutely no idea what to talk about with a girlfriend, so that ended after twenty-four hours. Two years later, the Litzes' younger daughter Essie had an engagement party to which our family was invited. When we arrived and I was told that Alice was there, I responded by running out to our car and spending the rest of the time hiding under the seat.

I had no idea that Alice went to Leeds until she was cast in the role of my older sister in *Mr. Fixit*. So there were Alice and I with leading roles in the Leeds play. I no longer had a crush on her, and I didn't know if she remembered me.

The play was a big success. I delivered my laugh lines well, thereby ensuring my fifteen minutes of fame.

Thankfully, neither Alice nor I mentioned the wedding.

Central High School

CENTRAL HIGH SCHOOL was the academic high school for boys in Philadelphia, and it was clear to my parents and counselor that I should go there. I, on the other hand, preferred coeducation, but the neighborhood high school had a deservedly poor reputation. Central High really was right for me. It was academically demanding, and the faculty was selected from the best teachers in the city. I don't imagine that the most elite of private schools had better. The students came from all over the city, from working- or middle-class families that were ambitious for their sons.

There was a regular class and an advanced class, which was for the smartest of the smart. I applied for the advanced class but was told that my IQ just wasn't high enough. That was okay. Those guys were truly gifted. Many went on to great careers, but I don't think they did better on average with their lives than the rest of us in the regular class. At reunions, many of the regular class students were now doctors, lawyers, or teachers, and the students from the advanced class were professors, computer types, and entrepreneurs who'd had varying degrees of success.

Of the many great teachers at Central High, one who stands out is Mr. B. He was my Spanish teacher for four of my eight terms of Spanish. He clearly loved his subject and his students, and though he was American, he spoke Spanish with a Spaniard's perfect Castilian accent. In upper-level classes he insisted that we speak only in Spanish, which was a very modern approach for high school at the time. The other teachers tended to treat language as an exercise in grammar and vocabulary. Mr. B. was a bit flamboyant in manner, and this always stoked the never-ending rumor mill about teachers' sexuality. Because I placed in AP Spanish, I only took one formal course in college. I'm not fluent, as my children and grandchildren (who are) will happily attest, but I've been conversant enough to communicate in the many Spanish-speaking countries I've visited and with the many Spanish-speaking patients I've treated.

The strongest department overall was English, and I remember one teacher after another who loved literature and loved to teach.

I had a number of neighborhood friends, one of whom, Bruce, suggested to me that I come over to meet a neighborhood kid named Rick. Bruce explained, "He's a great guy and he knows a lot of girls."

"Rick who?" I asked.

"Rick Blumberg."

Could this be the same guy who was constantly teased at Leeds?

It was indeed one and the same, but Rick turned out to be a really engaging and friendly guy. And he did know a lot of girls. There was often a party in his rec room on Saturday nights, and if there wasn't, he knew where one was. We played cards on Fridays, which was a great relief from the pressures of school. Rick became the center of our little high school social group, and we were all basically nerdy students, except for Rick; much to the frustration of his parents, Rick enjoyed socializing far too much to take school seriously. But he was a good person who was always loyal to his friends.

Rick's parents were lovely people. Jack, Rick's father, was a plainspoken, average-looking man who made a good living working long hours as a food broker, getting up in the middle hours of the night to buy fruits and vegetables, which he sold to the best restaurants in the city. His wife, Rick's mother, May, was quite a bit younger than Jack, and Rick was born before his mom was even out of her teens. She was headstrong and creative and quite a beautiful redhead. I think Jack must have wondered why it was that she went for him. May was beside herself as to why her son couldn't be more like his friends academically. Over the years, there was constant tension between Rick and his mom. I don't know how much this was about Rick's mannerisms or if it was really only about his school-work, but I know they bickered constantly. In those days teen-age boys were really never open or accepting about sexuality, except for making sneering references about "homos." Any who had such proclivities suffered in silence.

Mostly thanks to Rick, I had a dating life in high school, but I never had a real girlfriend. My parents insisted that I attend to studying, and going out during the week was not an option.

With me, relationships never lasted too long because of the "notches on the belt" mentality prevalent at the time (could it still be?). If a girl liked you, it was your prideful duty as a male to try to get as far as you could sexually (never mind what she—or you, for that matter—really wanted). It was then expected that you would tell all. I'm convinced that a lot of those clumsy attempts put an end to any possibility of really getting to know any number of pretty or interesting girls.

There was one girl in particular I never got to know in high school. Every morning I commuted to high school on a city bus, along with dozens of boys and girls. The boys were headed to Central High, and the girls were commuting to the neighboring Philadelphia High School for Girls (Girl's High). Some mornings there arrived a beautiful blond with long, straight hair down to her waist and a smile that melted my heart. She was always combing her hair and laughing with her girlfriends, and I developed a hopeless crush from afar. But my mornings were happier when she was on the bus. I asked a friend who she was and was informed "That's Fern Feinberg. Forget about her, Hoffman, you wouldn't stand a chance. She only dates seniors."

My first summer away from home was at age sixteen. I worked as a waiter at Camp Kennebec, a boys' camp for rich kids, in Waterville, Maine. Two of my friends had worked there the previous year. They got me the job, and I worked with them. It was eight weeks of what was practically slave labor. We worked seven days a week, waiting three meals, washing dishes, and doing all manner of painting and repairs for the princely sum of $125 for the summer along with room (a rustic cabin we all shared) and board (our food prepared by an old Irish cook of minimal culinary skills). He called me "camel driver," my camp nickname, because on the chilly Maine mornings I'd come to work in a hoodie, only my nose visible. I guess I was his idea of an Arab.

We waiters enjoyed each other's company, played sports, and had a lot of laughs and occasional fistfights. One of my friends was the head waiter, who had the job of waking us up in the morning. He must have thought he was a marine sergeant, because one morning he put his face right up to mine, yelling to get the hell up. He startled me, and though he was twice my size, I leapt up from the bed, put my face up to his, and screamed that if he ever did that again I would kill him. After that, the wake ups were more civilized.

We had a few adventures with the local girls. Female visitors were strictly forbidden on the campgrounds, but I had found myself a skinny little friend, and with the help of another waiter whose last name was Grosse, I smuggled her in, along with Grosse's date. The four of us found a hidden area for some kissing and cuddling, which is what we were doing when she turned to me and whispered, "I heard Grosse was a Jew." He wasn't. I answered, "He's not, but I am." She turned pale, but to her credit, she quickly got over it (maybe after looking for horns growing from my head and satisfying herself that I had none), and we returned to teen activities that were much better than talking.

It was probably the healthiest summer of my life, but I did not return to Camp Kennebec after that.

I wound up doing quite well at Central High, and my college boards were excellent but certainly not stratospheric. Because of this, my family, especially my mother's family from Massachusetts, vastly overestimated my chances of getting into what they referred to as a "prestige school."

My mother, her brother Irving, and my cousin Howard, who had gone to Williams College, all collaborated to fill out my applications and select the schools to which I'd apply. I had little say in the matter. Dad's contribution was to tell me to do what my mother said. I wrote essays on such things as my most formative intellectual experience, basically making things up. Howard's view was "It's all bullshit anyway." That was probably true, but bullshit wasn't my strong suit. After suffering through numerous visits and interviews, I can safely say that I was rejected by some of the most distinguished colleges and universities in the Northeast. The rejection that was the most gratuitously cruel came from Harvard, in a thick envelope. A thick envelope, of course, usually indicated acceptance because of the various enrollment forms included. Imagine my surprise when I opened it and found a rejection letter, along with an article of many pages titled "What to Do When You Don't Get into the College of Your Choice."

I'm sure the pompous sadists at the Harvard admissions office had a few snickers coming up with that.

I was admitted to Penn and to Franklin and Marshall College (F&M), the latter being a small men's college in Lancaster, Pennsylvania, with a good reputation for science and premed. I believed, correctly, that I'd fare better at a small school, so off to F&M I headed that fall.

How did I decide on premed? I first learned that I was premed at about the age of ten. It was during one of the summers my family and I spent in Gloucester, crowding into Uncle Irving's tiny one-bedroom apartment for a week or just a weekend. My cousins Howard and David (who waited tables in Gloucester during the summers) were also staying there. My mother, my brother, and I would all pile into his living room, sleeping on the sofa bed or futons on the floor. We loved it, and I think Irving loved having us too.

One evening we were sitting around, and Irving was feeling mellow after his scotch. He took me on his lap and said, "Jeffrey, I know you are a good student, and coming from this family, you can go on to be anything you want. Now which medical specialty are you planning on?"

Everybody else thought it was hilarious, but I wasn't so sure.

Irving was the family success, though, and therefore, to my mother, he was the authority on everything. He was a gifted lawyer and did very well, especially after World War II, but he'd struggled a lot when he was getting started in the 1930s. He was of the opinion that it made no sense for any smart Jewish boy to pursue anything but medicine, a sure road to wealth and respect. He had been educated at Boston University and the Boston University School of Law. According to the family story, because his father had been a cobbler who lost his business in the Great Depression, he could not afford to send Irving to Harvard, and Irving had to settle for Boston University.

He never got over that, and I suppose my family didn't either.

College Days

In 1962, Franklin and Marshall College (F&M) was a small, pretty campus full of leafy trees and ivy-covered Victorian buildings, with a steepled chapel and a mixture of modern and older dorms. It seemed welcoming, and when I arrived, ready to live away from home for a second time (the first, of course, being Camp Kennebec in Maine), I was happy to be there. My fellow freshmen seemed similar enough to boys (it was not yet coed then) I had known in high school that I did not feel out of place. It was apparent, however, that many were from well-to-do families. The most serious students among us were the premeds and prelaws, strivers who aspired to comfortable upper-middle-class lives. F&M specialized in us.

There was a small contingent of local students, even a few commuters. They were mostly math and science majors, and they were the brightest of us. F&M was a very good college but not necessarily a highly competitive one when it came to admissions. There were many there who drank and played their way through their four undergraduate years, generally majoring in business or sociology. English was also a favored and rigorous major, and many students with interests in the arts, drama, or journalism were drawn to it. The Green Room, the college drama club, gave birth to a few successful acting careers, Treat Williams and Roy Scheider among the most prominent.

F&M was a haven for bright Ivy League rejects, a quintessential "safety school" whose students' résumés showed that they were excellent students but whose total packages were not quite distinguished enough to interest the top-tier schools. We were well aware of this, and it was the subject of interminable obsessing in freshman dorm bull sessions.

My freshman roommate was a prematurely jaded self-styled sophisticate from a wealthy North Jersey family. He found me hopelessly naive and was determined to take me under his wing. "Hoffman, Hoffman, you just don't get it," he'd tell me as he condescended to lecture me and share his profundities about women, politics, or religion. At the time of John F. Kennedy's assassination I was a sophomore, and like most of the world, I was devastated. I shared this with my roommate, and he rolled his eyes, looking bored and impatient. "Hoffman," he told me, "a year from now everyone will have forgotten about it." He was really a lost, directionless soul. He eventually dropped out of college and emigrated to Canada to avoid the draft.

There was a classmate named Joe, a skinny, unhealthy-looking guy who came from a small town in South Jersey. He constantly whined about how poorly his small-town high school had prepared him for college and that he barely understood his classes and didn't expect to make it past the first semester. We genuinely felt sorry for him until his first semester 4.0 (straight A's). After his second semester 4.0, we started calling him 4.0 Joe. Of course, he graduated Phi Beta Kappa and later Alpha Omega Alpha at Penn Med.

The first year was relatively easy for me. I was well prepared at Central High and got almost all A's, doing especially well in freshman chemistry, a subject that stumped and eliminated half the premeds.

Because of our "Ivy League envy," many of us considered transferring to other colleges. The was a rumor that if you did well your first year, you might be able to get in somewhere that wouldn't accept you right out of high school. The college, possibly panicked about the potential hemorrhage of its best students, came up with a plan to tempt us to remain, the College Scholar Program. The freshmen with the highest grade-point averages were invited to participate in this new and exclusive group. Members did not have to declare a major or have the usual distribution requirements, and they could take any course in any department they chose. Your grades were honors pass or fail. Also, a special seminar room—and later an entire building—was designated for college scholars only, where special seminars were provided. When I was invited, how could I resist?

As the years passed, I came to the realization that though I was a pretty good student, I was not much of a scholar.

The first seminar, the course "Free Will versus Determinism" was actually pretty interesting, with readings from various existentialists, behaviorists, and other -ists that stimulated a lot of late-night discussions. I guess that's what college is supposed to be about. Some of the other seminars, on topics such as Eastern religions and philosophy of science, sounded good in theory but demanded the reading of original texts. A lot of it was tedious to me, and I couldn't bring myself to learn the material just for the sake of learning, which was probably obvious to the seminar professors.

I did get to choose some great electives, especially in English and political science. I took classes in international politics, political theory, the modern novel, and modern poetry that exposed me to books and ideas more expansive than anything in high school.

I also took the requisite premed courses and the required courses for a chem major, a subject in which I initially did well. By the time I reached upper-level classes, though, I found that I wasn't all that interested in chemistry either. I had a roommate a year ahead of me who eventually took a PhD in physical chemistry at the Massachusetts Institute of

Technology. It was clear how much he loved the subject, and I knew the difference.

However, my elementary knowledge of chemistry did have a real practical value in my family's history.

Hoffman's Delicatessen had been failing since the death of Nana a few years before. She was a sweet little Yiddish lady who was loved by everyone. She was also a spectacularly good kosher cook, and whatever she was making for the day was the special at the store. The patrons were crazy about her, and everyone called her "Mom." I was close to Nana, who spoiled me. On many occasions she was a human body shield, protecting me from the assaults of my father. She died at the age of sixty-five from a heart attack. It was devastating for all of us. After that the business went downhill, despite Zeda's attempts to carry on and do the cooking himself. It just wasn't the same.

When the store closed a few years later, my father and grandfather got a little money for the property on Twenty-Ninth Street, but that was all. My father got a series of low-paying jobs, the last of which was as a housing inspector for the City of Philadelphia. This involved going into the worst neighborhoods in the city in order to inspect and list the slum landlord's housing violations. I once asked Dad if he was afraid to go into those neighborhoods. "Not at all," he replied. "They know I'm their friend."

So, Mother had to become our main breadwinner. She was a teacher of dental assisting in the Philadelphia public schools. Her own degree was in dental hygiene, earned many years before at Temple University. To keep her job, she had to get a bachelor's degree followed by a master's degree and then a master's degree plus thirty credits for pay raises. But her plans were almost stillborn due to the chemistry requirement she had to pass as a science teacher.

She was desperate, and she was failing. No pass, no BA; no BA, no teaching job.

Her son the chemistry major was expected to come to the rescue, and many weekends of torture followed. Mother was a bright and energetic woman, but basic chemistry, particularly the math parts, eluded her.

"Mother, these chem equations, they're no different than algebra."

"I hope you're not saying that to make me feel better." It was the most brutal C she ever earned, but she made it through, and so did our family.

As college scholars, we were required to do an honors project in any subject we chose. I decided to do a paper on D. H. Lawrence's poetry, a decision pretty much based entirely on my enjoyment of a course in modern poetry. It turned out to be a gruesome mistake.

You may wonder why, with my academic interests and enthusiasms, I was a premed at all. As I mentioned earlier, the only acceptable professions for a smart Jewish boy in my family's view were medicine and law. It was inconceivable that a boy who had the intellectual capacity to pursue medicine would do otherwise. As a teen, it would have been futile for me to argue. But I also had other influences. My cousin Howard, who is ten years my senior, had been an unabashed premed with a degree from Williams College. A charming guy with average looks, he had a way with women that I enviously attempted to emulate. He was not intellectually brilliant, but he was persistent, energetic, and competitive. He went on to have an extremely successful career in neurosurgery and medical entrepreneurship, making millions on a variety of projects involving MRI machines, PET Scanners, and rehab hospitals for himself and his partners, myself included to a limited extent.

I admired Howard, and he took to me. While I was a premed, he was a neurosurgical resident at Columbia, and he was my host in New York City for a number of memorable weekends. He took me on his morning rounds in his resident whites, and I thought it was the coolest thing in the world. Howard's enthusiasm was infectious. His life was neurosurgery and having his way with as many nurses as possible. That seemed pretty good to me.

I realized quickly that doctors get a lot of respect and made good money and that once I got to be a med student, I might even get more dates. I didn't think so much about the hard work.

Try not to conclude that these were shallow considerations. To a nineteen-year-old, they were perfectly sound (to a seventy-two-year-old too).

At F&M, we were exposed to the sort of platitudes that encourage you to follow your passion. But what if, like many undergraduates, you really don't have one? I had a fraternity brother, Mark, who was originally a premed and an excellent one. He was editor in chief of the college newspaper, switched to prelaw, and went on to Harvard Law School. I remember having a long conversation with him about why he made the change. I don't remember what he said specifically, but I recall that he was decisive. I briefly considered going with prelaw or journalism, but in the end I stuck with premed, and it turned out to be a good choice. Or maybe I lacked Mark's courage.

In most premed programs the make-or-break course was organic chemistry, but at F&M at the time, most of the premed bodies were buried in invertebrate zoology, taught by a sadist named James MacManus (Jimmy Mac). He seemed to take pleasure in the early-term aborting of the careers of aspiring docs. He always returned exams in grade order, highest first, watching the students squirm like his beloved worms. I studied hard, did poorly, and got a pass.

Another required premed course was comparative anatomy and embryology, taught by a popular professor, Harry Lane. It required brute memorization, a skill definitely needed in med school. At the end of the first semester we dissected a cat, and we were permitted—encouraged actually—to bring the cat home to study for the final. Not wanting to fall behind the others, I packed my formaldehyde-soaked cat in an oilcloth and sack and deposited it in the family rec room, intending to use it to study over the weekend. We had a cleaning lady named Hattie at the time who had been with our family for many years and came on Saturdays.

That Saturday morning our family was awakened by a shriek that may have been heard in Lancaster. When I looked outside, there was Hattie running down Lynnewood Road screaming for help from Jesus.

In our rec room, my little cat's head was peeking out of its sack. My parents tried to contact Hattie to beg her to come back, swearing that we weren't involved in voodoo, but we never heard from Hattie again.

The College Scholar Program grading system wasn't hard to figure out. An A in the class was an honors; anything else was pass (except, God forbid, fail). At the end of the semester you got a progress letter, and the wording of the four-honor, three-honor, two-honor, one-honor (you're in trouble), and zero-honor (bye-bye) letters were always the same. As the years went by the quality of my letters slowly diminished, and after two one-honor letters in a row, I was booted from the College Scholars Program at the start of my second semester, senior year. In my defense, my grade point average would have been pretty good if it had just been letter grades. So, second semester of senior year, no longer a college scholar, I still had my thesis to complete on the poetry of D. H. Lawrence, so at least I had a shot at graduating with honors.

My first thesis adviser was a psoriatic and very minor poet who was a visiting professor that year. My subject, D. H. Lawrence, was pretty interesting, and I enjoyed reading his work and the works of his major influences, most notably Thomas Hardy. The writing of the paper, however, was pure torture.

The psoriatic poet left the college abruptly and was replaced by Andy Card, a kindly and encouraging man who helped me through the ordeal that followed.

On the day I was to defend my paper, the entire English Department was present in a small seminar room. Also present was Professor Samuel Hines, a guest interrogator from Swarthmore College who happened to be a world authority on Thomas Hardy. I was naturally a little anxious, but I felt that I knew my subject well and was fairly confident going in. I'm sure the English Department was a little skittish too, wondering how the *ex*–college scholar would do in front of Swarthmore guy. When it was time to ask the first question, they deferred to him.

"So, Mr. Hoffman, tell us. What is a poem?"

I would have done better with a question about the implications of the Schrödinger wave equation (a lot better, actually). This was a question that any half-facile English major could have come up with a half-facile answer to. Not me. I froze, clueless. I have no idea how long the humiliating silence lasted. In retrospect, I still don't know if it was a fair question or a stupid one, but the rest of the questioning was moot. I was able to defend details of the paper, but I did less well the further afield the questioning went. It was apparent that I was no English major. So, no honors, no college scholar.

Fortunately, F&M wasn't just about academic stress. It had a healthy fraternity system to provide distraction, friendship, and release of pressure, especially on weekends. There were thirteen fraternity houses, each of which had its own personality and ethnic or religious makeup. There were fraternities that specialized in Catholics, Protestants (upper class), preppie types, self-anointed intellectuals, and alcohol majors. Most of the Jewish boys were drawn to either Zeta Beta Tau (ZBT), the place for well-to-do and socially ambitious Jewish boys, or Pi Lambda Phi (Pi Lamb), which was an eclectic mixture of

Jews, blacks, and iconoclasts. Other fraternities called Pi Lamb "the United Nations," which was not meant as a compliment.

For me, Pi Lamb was the only choice. I got drunk for the first time at one of its rush parties, and I loved the place. My father wouldn't let me pledge as a freshman, fearing that it would be a disruption to my studies and would ruin my grades. When I did very well my freshman year, he reluctantly let me pledge as a first-semester sophomore.

The rituals—even the hazing, silly as it was—bonded us, and the fraternity was a place where you felt at home and accepted. Our parties were raucous and were generally considered the best on campus. The music was mostly Motown, control of the selection process jealously guarded by the black brothers. For some reason I remember "Foot Stompin'" by the Flares, when we made the floorboards vibrate and the rafters shake, and "Stubborn Kind of Fellow" by Marvin Gaye, just because I like Marvin Gaye.

At the end of each party the brothers would form an intoxicated circle, arms around each other, and sing a fraternity song called "Jolly Laddies" to the tune of "Tavern in the Town." Hokey but fun.

During rush periods we would sit around, self-importantly smoking cigars and evaluating prospective pledges. At rush parties, we would dress in our best three-piece suits and tell jokes or give speeches extolling the virtues of Pi Lamb.

I was a decent speaker and did this every year. We competed for the best students, athletes, political types, or just people we liked and didn't want to lose to the hated Zeebs (of ZBT). My job on rush committee was to recruit college scholars. I think we got one after me.

A most intense effort surrounded pledging period, intended to mold allegiance to the fraternity mostly through a series of hazing rituals, some humiliating, some silly, with enforced push-ups, dorm raids, and obedience to any brother who craved a pizza at three o'clock in the morning. When I was pledging I oddly found it all pretty funny, and I'd break out laughing when screamed at, earning me more push-ups.

The pledging period culminated in Hell Week, which was actually a long weekend of creative sadism. The pledges were kept sleep-deprived most of the weekend, with the intended purpose being the breakdown of all barriers to self, causing surrender to the brotherhood. I'm sure there were more than a few real psychotic breaks during this now mostly outlawed process of fraternity torment.

On the final night, pledges were instructed to stare at a burning candle while listening to a repetitive Bach fugue and contemplating their answer to the "final test."

"Give ten reasons why you want to join Pi Lambda Phi."

Then, exhausted and confused, the pledge was escorted into the "interrogation room." Standing behind him was his pledge father, an older brother who had been his personal mentor during the pledge period and was now there to "support" him. The pledge would be made to stare at a bright lamp, and the questioning went something like this:

Inquisitor: "Pledge, I have to tell you, you have been one of the worst pledges in the history of Pi Lamb. You were almost blackballed last week."

Pledge Father: "But he really wants to be a brother. He'll do anything. Just give him a chance." (The pledge's lips quiver.)

Inquisitor: "Okay, pledge, this is your last chance. Have you come up with your ten reasons?"

Pledge (discerning a glimmer of hope): "Well, the brothers are great. The house is nice, the food is great, the parties are the best—"

Inquisitor (interrupting loudly): "What! What? We don't need you to tell us what's great about Pi Lamb! Give your ten reasons why Pi Lamb should take you!"

Pledge (pathetically whining): "But I thought you said to give ten reasons why I wanted to join Pi Lamb!"

Inquisitor: "You idiot! Weren't you even listening!"

By reason two, if he gets that far, the pledge is reduced to a weeping puddle of Jell-O.

Inquisitor: "Alright, just get him out of my sight."

The pledge father then tries a desperate intervention.

Pledge Father: "You've got to give him a chance. What about the 'trial by fire'?"

Silence in the room.

Inquisitor: "You can't be serious. We haven't done that in years. We could go to jail."

Pledge: "I'll do it!"

The pledge was then hustled into another room, where his pants were removed. A fake branding iron with the Greek letters Pi Lambda Phi was waved before him, and then a red-hot fork was pressed against a pizza for a sizzling sound.

And that was it. The poor broken pledge passed into brotherhood. Silly? Sadistic? Dangerous? Yeah, but it was fun!

In the junior and senior years, a premed's preoccupation—obsession, really—was about getting into med school and which med school. A large percentage of the students were from the Philadelphia area, so many applied to the local medical schools. There was the Philadelphia College of Osteopathy (better to go to dental school), Hahnemann (which was rumored to be struggling to keep its accreditation), Temple (a very good and respected school), and Jefferson Medical College (excellent, with a reputation of grinding its students to dust). But the crème de la crème was the University of Pennsylvania, where no more than two or three F&M students were admitted each year. To younger premeds, seniors who got into Penn were like heroes. Med school was expensive, and as a lark I applied to the Pennsylvania Medical

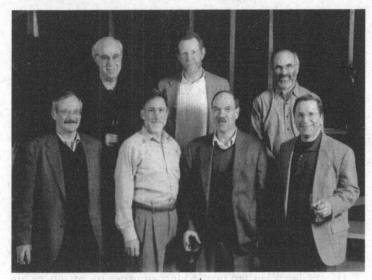

Pi Lamb Brothers 35ᵗʰ F&M Reunion

Society, which gave a few full tuition scholarships to Pennsylvania residents.

I applied to Penn and several other schools. Because there were so many applicants from F&M, admissions people from Penn came to our campus to interview us all in one afternoon. I went to the interview decked out in my trusty three-piece gray interview suit, and it seemed to go reasonably well. The only bit of encouragement I got was that I was told that my MCATs were very good. I really did not expect to get accepted, and I was deliriously happy to get the good news when it came. As it turned out, a record number of F&M students were admitted to Penn our year: about a dozen, four times the usual. Professor William Kennedy, dean of admissions at Penn, and Professor James Darlington, the premed adviser at F&M, were personal friends and were both said to be retiring that year. The inflated number of admissions was rumored to be a retirement kiss.

Penn was relatively expensive, but Mother and Dad told me not to worry about that. They said they would "beg, borrow, or steal" to pay for it.

The competition for the scholarships from the Pennsylvania Medical Society included the top premeds in the state, and only five or six scholarships would be awarded. I had just been booted from the College Scholars Program, a negative distinction. For some stupid reason, I felt compelled to inform the medical society about this and did so by letter.

A few weeks later I got a letter from the Pennsylvania Medical Society asking if I would accept the scholarship if offered, which I assumed was a form letter sent to all applicants.

I used my home address for all official correspondence, and when another letter arrived the following week, my parents asked if they could open it. I was planning on coming home that weekend, and I insisted that they wait until I was present.

So, early Friday evening as I was walking down Lynnewood Road and reaching sight of my house, Dad stood in the doorway reading the letter loud enough for several neighbors to conclude that he'd gone berserk. I'd been awarded a full-tuition scholarship. I was embarrassed but understood my parents' pride and excitement.

To this day I have no idea how I got that scholarship. Maybe they figured that anyone dumb enough to send them that letter about getting booted out of the College Scholars Program needed all the help he could get.

Penn Med and Internship

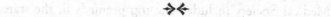

THE CLASS OF 1970 at Penn Med consisted mostly of men (there were about 6 women in a class of 125). They were a good-looking group, taken mostly from Ivy League schools and the top small colleges, along with 1 or 2 of the best pre-meds from each of the local colleges in the Philadelphia area. They were very bright, and many were clearly brilliant, but I remember not really being too intimidated academically. I personally felt well prepared for med school by F&M, and it soon became obvious that most were feeling as overwhelmed by the demands of med school as I was.

Socially I was somewhat more intimidated, feeling that many were somehow more polished and confident than me. I tended to keep to myself and didn't really make any close friends while I was a med student.

Even though I had a tuition scholarship, living on campus was costly, so I took a job as a dorm counselor to freshman undergraduates, for which I received room and board. The freshmen on my floor were pretty boisterous, and I didn't do too well controlling them. They were a distraction that didn't enhance my studies. I trudged daily that first semester to my gross anatomy class, where we dissected Ernest (you always named your cadaver). We said that we were work-ing in dead Ernest (get it?). The sheer volume of material we needed to learn was beyond anything I'd ever experienced in college, and I felt the need to study constantly just to keep up. Nevertheless, I got my best preclinical grade—a B—from Ernest along with histology and neuroanatomy.

Biochemistry, physiology, pathology, molecular biology, pharmacology, and other subjects followed. Besides requiring even greater amounts of brute memorization, these courses were often more conceptually challenging. I worked hard and managed to get mediocre grades. And like most med students, I came down with symptoms of many of the diseases described in nauseating detail in pathology, the results of which were dramatically demonstrated at required-attendance autopsies. I somehow recall the postmortem of a frail middle-aged woman whose internal organs were riddled with cancer. She had a beautiful, delicate face that retained the expression of horrible suffering she must have worn at the end. Of course, cancer was the disease I was most sure I was developing (everybody had their favorite). Later as a third-year student I was occasionally involved in the treatment of patients my own age who in fact did have cancer, and my identification with them was at times excruciating.

By the way, all that stuff about young, brave cancer victims that you see on TV is pretty much bullshit. They are just as scared as you or I might be in those circumstances, often in denial and sometimes very obnoxious.

It was all pretty exhausting, yet trotting off to the med school in my little white jacket from the dorms made me feel proud. The med students were the most esteemed and envied at the university. Only a small number of premeds from the undergraduate school made it to the med school there.

Being located on the university campus made it possible to participate in the cultural and social amenities of a great university, even if only occasionally. Once in a while I ran into an acquaintance from the past in the hospital or on campus, and wearing the white jacket made me feel like a big deal. There was one fellow I'd gone to Hebrew school with, a brilliant student back then and at Penn, where he was doing graduate studies in Middle Eastern languages. While I was impressed that I was a med student, to his credit, I don't think that he was in the slightest.

As a dorm counselor, I sometimes arranged mixers for my freshmen with the freshmen women. I had a friend, a law student and fellow impoverished dorm counselor, and we tried to set up social gatherings for diversion. We'd gather her freshmen and my freshman into some party space. The mixers were awkward, but we tried.

The stress of the early med school years took its toll, and I developed colitis, a stress-related ailment that has remained a little token of my med school experience.

I went out with the occasional undergrad but had little time or inclination to pursue anything serious. There was another med school in Philadelphia, the Women's Medical College of Pennsylvania, where I attended a social and met an Israeli student who was a lieutenant in the Israel Defense Forces and as prickly a cactus flower as any Sabra. Though she was a year behind me in school, she was a couple of years older. She often accused me of being "such a boy." I'm not sure why, but I suppose she was right.

When I had graduated from college, my mother's father, Grampy George, had given me a gift of a thousand dollars. My parents urged me to save it, which I did, but only until the summer of 1967, when I spent it on my first trip to Europe with my friend Rick Blumberg. It was the days of hippiedom, and Europe was crowded with kids from all over the world, hitchhiking here and there, smoking a lot of strange substances, and generally having a good time. I was woefully disorganized and managed to loose my passport and Eurail pass more than once, thereby requiring much travel by thumb.

Rick and I covered a lot of ground that summer: London, Paris, Madrid, Barcelona, the running of the bulls at Pamplona, the Costa Brava, Rome (with a performance of *Aida* at the Baths), Switzerland, Austria, Germany, Holland, and Denmark. We landed in London, which at the time seemed like another planet, with strange accents and tiny houses. In Pamplona, Rick really did run with the bulls while I waited safely in a doorway. We attended a bullfight, which was colorful but as brutal as you'd imagine. The Spaniards loved it, and I was mesmerized. In Copenhagen, they told us never to pronounce it "Copenhahgen" because that was how the Germans said it, and they still hated the Germans.

There was a song called "Puppet on a String" that had won a European song competition that year and was played all over Europe. A catchy tune, it was kind of the theme song of the trip, and when I remember the summer of 1967 that song always comes to mind.

It was relatively cheap to travel. Youth hostels cost fifty cents per night, and you could stay at a decent hotel for between two and five dollars. I had a brief encounter with a British girl in Sitges, which is on the coast near Barcelona. It was in a ruins overlooking a beach. The area was heavily patrolled by the Guardia Civil, Francisco Franco's very nasty police force. If we had been caught, we could easily have been shot in this very Catholic country.

In Germany while hitchhiking on the Autobahn, Rick and I got tired and decided to snooze on the side of the highway. About an hour later, we were awakened by the German Highway Patrol shining flashlights in our faces. They looked like storm troopers, but instead of sending us to concentration camps, they let us go after checking our passports.

We were soon picked up by a couple of German girls, one of whom was a very cute freckled English teacher who assured me that she really liked Jewish guys. She more or less proved it during the day we spent together on Scheveningen Beach in Holland.

We covered a lot of ground that summer, with minimal sleep and minimal cash. It was a well-spent one thousand dollars.

After the ordeal of the preclinical years, we all looked forward to dealing with actual patients. My first rotation was pediatrics, and I spent one of the months on the cancer ward at the Children's Hospital of Philadelphia (CHOP). These were children dying of various gruesome cancers—leukemia mostly—and it was the saddest innocent suffering I've

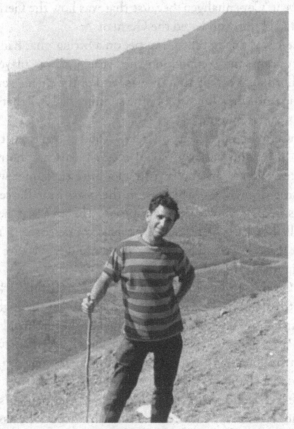

Rambling through Europe

ever seen. Because it was a research hospital, the kids were often subjected to harsh research protocols involving multiple blood drawings, lumbar punctures, or other painful procedures, with little benefit. They mostly died, but I know that future victims of childhood leukemia benefited.

The most dreaded third-year rotation was internal medicine on Ward B, the women's ward at the Hospital of the University of Pennsylvania (HUP). Notoriously harsh, it was run by Dr. William Williams, hematologist and hard-ass.

On my first day on Ward B, I had the misfortune of having to present the first case. It was a patient who presented with severe chest pain.

Standing before my terrified third-year classmates, I was asked the differential diagnosis (causes) of chest pain. There are many structures in the human chest capable of causing pain, and that morning I was able to remember very few of them. Before long Dr. Williams asked me to sit down, and I did, in a puddle of sweat and failure. The others were just relieved that they weren't me.

Nevertheless, I worked hard through the rest of the rotation, and my next presentation was much better. At the end of the two months, Dr. Williams called each of us into his office for our evaluation. He acknowledged that after my initial disaster I had worked really hard, and I earned a C for the rotation. He helpfully assured me that if I continued my effort I would make an adequate internist, which was probably his way of encouraging me to find another specialty. His assessment was accurate, and I actually took it as a compliment. His standard of adequacy was quite high. But to this day I can give the differential diagnosis of chest pain as well as any internist.

Rotations in surgery, ob-gyn, psychiatry, and briefer subspecialty rotations followed. I considered neurology (a highly intellectually precise and fascinating specialty), obstetrics (where we third-year students delivered many babies and did all the circumcisions), psychiatry, and yes, even internal medicine as possible career choices. My psychiatry rotation assignment was at the Institute of the Pennsylvania Hospital, one of the most highly regarded psychiatric treatment centers and the oldest in the country. Even as a third-year student, I felt an affinity for this specialty. The third-year rotation was led by Dr. Newell Fischer, a puckish and very smart psychoanalyst who was a wonderful and encouraging teacher. He went on to be, among other things, a president of the American Psychoanalytic Association.

The following summer (1968), Rick and I decided to take another trip together. For some reason, we thought it would be neat to spend the month of August driving to Mexico City and Acapulco. Rick's father foolishly lent us his station wagon for this dubious venture. On the way down we drove through the Deep South, a place where liberal Yankee Jewish boys were not exactly welcome. We stopped in an old country store in rural Alabama, where a middle-aged country boy dressed in American Gothic was the proprietor. It didn't take long for Rick and Country Boy to get into it on politics. Rick identified himself as a Eugene McCarthy guy, and of course Country Boy was for George Wallace.

In a sudden non sequitur, Country Boy asked, "You boys are Jews, ain't yuh?" Rick answered perfectly. "My parents are Jews, but I'm an atheist." Country Boy said, "You boys just wait here a minute." And then he went into the back of the store. "Rick," I said. "He's getting his shotgun! Let's go!" Rick was smart enough to agree, and we didn't wait to find out if I was right.

We drove on through Mississippi, Louisiana, and Texas on the way to Mexico. At one point we saw a black teenager hitchhiking on the highway, and Rick wanted to pick him up. I refused, reasoning that if any cracker saw the three of us riding together, they'd mistake us for Freedom Riders and lynch us. Freedom Riders were mostly youths from the North who came south to help blacks in civil rights demonstrations, including sit-ins at restaurants that refused to serve them. They were not welcome by all southerners, and some had been lynched by the Ku Klux Klan.

So, we parked and waited at the side road, probably scaring the teenager half to death. The dispute ended when a black truck driver stopped and picked him up.

We drove hundreds of miles through the beautiful mountains of Mexico. Fortunately for us our car functioned well, as the mountains were full of bad hombres who would have happily murdered a couple of gringos for the contents of their car and wallets.

I don't recall much about our time in Mexico City except that it was one vast, unregulated traffic jam. We were stopped once by a cop for an unspecified traffic violation, but he let us go for a "fine" of three dollars.

Rural Mexico had as many stray dogs as people, and unfortunately, on the way to Acapulco I hit and killed one of them. I got out of the car and waited a few minutes, and when no one showed up, I suggested that we get going. But Rick, who was and is a dog lover, unconvinced that the dog was just an unfortunate stray, insisted that we try to find the owner. Lo and behold, a few minutes later appeared three Mexican boys, tears flowing as they babbled in rapid-fire Spanish about their beloved dog. I explained in my high school Spanish how sorry we were but that it was an accident and we hadn't seen the dog. The tears continued to flow until I got it. I reached for my wallet and gave then each three dollars. The tears disappeared, and off they ran.

The little shakedown artists probably threw the dog in front of the car.

We spent a few days in Acapulco, saw the famous Cliff Divers, and went to an authentic local bullfight. We also went to a local beach where a hippie offered us some Acapulco Gold.

Rick loved it, but I got psychotic and hallucinated all night. I thought I was going to die and begged to be taken to a hospital. The hippie said that going to the hospital would only land me in jail, so we spent the night on the beach, where Rick did a stellar job calming me down over the coming hours. I had tried marijuana once or twice before, but the Acapulco Gold was unbelievably strong, and I wasn't ready for its effect. Fortunately I was with Rick, who was really my only experienced pot-smoking friend.

Finally heading home, Rick and I were adventured out. I had to get back to med school and he to his high school teaching, and we drove as fast as we could mostly taking turns, with one of us at the wheel while the other slept in the car. I was driving on the Kentucky Turnpike in the early morning hours, the car loaded with souvenirs, when I had a sudden rear-tire blowout. I completely lost control of the car, which swerved all over the highway. Fortunately, there was no other traffic at the time. We crashed into a concrete bridge abutment. Miraculously, I walked out of the car uninjured, and Rick had no more than a twisted ankle. But the car was totaled. Rick insisted that I call his father, mainly to explain that the accident was my fault. I stammered during a long-distance call to Mr. Blumberg. "Uh, Mr. Blumberg, it's Jeff. The good news is that we're all right." We flew home from Louisville.

The fourth year for med students at Penn was essentially an elective year. It was also the most fun year of my life. After three years as a dorm counselor, I finally moved into an apartment off campus, which I shared with a fraternity brother from F&M and a guy from Swarthmore who was hardly ever there. My electives were classes chosen for the purpose of narrowing down my career choices or were review electives so that I could hone skills that, I thought, I would need to lessen my chances of killing someone during my upcoming internship.

I took cardiology to read EKGs, radiology for basic X-rays, and a month of junior internship, where you basically functioned as an intern under the very close supervision of a medical resident. I also took electives in neurology and ob-gyn to get a better feel for those specialties.

But I fell in love with psychiatry while working in the Adolescent Unit. The Adolescent Unit, also at the Institute of the Pennsylvania Hospital, was an inpatient unit for very ill teenagers: manic-depressives, schizophrenics, severely self-destructive borderlines, and any number of addicts, mostly involving heroin. Many of the patients were not much younger than I was. I'm sure I overidentified with them and underestimated how sick most of them were. Some of the addicts were charming and probably psychopathic. And some of the female patients were kind of cute. I'm not sure how much I learned about adolescent psychiatry, but after those two months I knew that I wanted to be a psychiatrist. It was also the only course in med school in which I got an honors, so my professors must have seen something in me too.

I joined the med school psychiatric society, also known as the future shrinks club, and one of the volunteer activities was something called "Talking Points." The idea was that other students would be able to chat with Penn Med students, who would be stationed in various places on the Penn campus, about any little problem—as though having the white jacket qualified us to deal with anything. But we were given referral resources and a little training about recognizing if a problem was beyond our pay grade.

Lucky me, I was stationed in a small room in the basement of the undergraduate women's dorm. The main purpose of the "patients" who showed up was to check me out, and the interest was mutual. I don't think I lost any undergraduates to mental illness, but whether I did anybody any good is debatable.

I had plenty of free time during that fourth year, and so having my own apartment was timely, and I had lots of friendly female companionship that year.

I guess that now that I was a senior med student, women may finally have taken the long view and seen a future in me. There were lots of little flings and one not so little one with a very nice nurse who loved me and whom I treated badly. I still regret that and hope that she has had a wonderful life.

I chose an internship in Washington, DC, at the Washington Hospital Center, the most important criterion being a call schedule of every fourth night, which was better than the usual every third night or, God forbid, every other night. It was called a mixed medical internship, which was similar to today's transitional medical internship. These are internships designed for individuals who are not going into internal medicine. My internship included several months of medicine and several months of electives. The internship year was not included in psychiatry residencies, which were then three years.

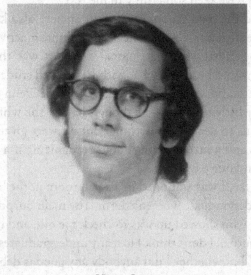

Hippie Intern

The internship turned out to be of very good quality, and my internship year was better and more fun than that year is supposed to be.

If you are not frightened to death when you start as an intern, you are in the wrong profession. If you are lucky, you come out feeling like a doctor.

For the first time you are called on to make decisions, often in the middle of the night when you are the first to evaluate a new patient or respond to a middle-of-the-night emergency on your floor.

The decision sometimes came down to "should I start a treatment I'm not totally sure about, thereby risking the patient's life," or "should I call the resident, waking him with a question and risking his wrath for interrupting his sleep with something that by now I should know the answer to."

During the numerous elective months, I took night call in the emergency room (ER) and over the year learned to manage a number of sometimes complex medical emergencies on my own.

My first rotation as an intern was in the ER, and my first case was a guy with acute urinary obstruction. Somehow I recalled the technique learned in a urology rotation of putting a Foley catheter through a swollen prostate, and lo and behold, the urine streamed out, much to the relief of my very grateful patient. I thought to myself "Hey, this intern stuff isn't so tough after all."

Over the year I learned to manage other things. Acute pulmonary edema? Gastrointestinal bleed? Diabetic ketoacidosis? Bring it on!

As an intern I often hung out with two guys, Steve Quint and Len Seeve, who were also future psychiatrists. I suppose we shared a certain outlook, perhaps irreverence, that drew us to each other and helped us get through the trials of internship. This was a time of unrest among young people in general, and whenever the interns had a beef with the administration, you could be sure that Len, the rebel among us, was in the middle of it.

Once we were called into the medical director's office about some dispute over night call, and the director threatened to fire us. I, of course, caved immediately, but this only stoked Len's indignation further. Fortunately, we all made it through the internship.

I lost track of Quint, but Len and his wife Carine, who became a pathologist, and Fern and I have remained friends for life.

Just before I moved to Washington, DC, a female friend commented to me that she had a girlfriend who was teaching there and maybe I'd like to ask her out. Her name was Fern Feinberg.

I thought to myself, "There can't be too many Fern Feinbergs." She had to be the one I'd had a silent crush on in high school, the girl who only dated seniors. Now that I was a young doctor, I figured that was at least as good as being a senior and that she'd go out with me.

So, on June 30, the night before my internship started, instead of staying home not sleeping, I went out with Fern on our first date. I shared my anxieties with her over a lobster dinner. We ate at an upscale restaurant, and I ordered Maine lobster. I dropped a large morsel and quickly bent under the table, hoping that Fern wouldn't notice. Okay, it was a little disgusting, but I considered lobster meat precious. I have yet to hear the end of this gauche little display, but somehow she continued going out with me anyway.

It was, of course, one and the same Fern, and we dated throughout the year. We had a great time, and she laughed at my lame jokes. After not too long I knew that she was the girl for me, and she felt the same way. How did I know that she was the girl for me? In a way you could say that we had an arranged marriage, except it was Fern and I who arranged it. I was always sensitive about being "controlled" by women, probably in reaction to a rather controlling mother. I was also really averse to women who seemed spoiled or entitled. Fern grew up in a lower-middle-class household like me and seemed really appreciative of things. She was a great teacher, and she was conscientious to a fault. I knew that she would be a loyal and good wife. She has often commented that she wished she were more self-confident or that she'd had more guidance from her parents, but guidance can cut both ways. She was smart, and we shared similar values. We have been a great and complementary team. Oh, yes—and she was gorgeous. All this may not sound Hollywood romantic, and maybe it wasn't. But I know that we love and need each other, more now than ever. I'm the strategic planner in our lives while she is the detail person, but we always have made big decisions together.

Fern grew up in Philadelphia, the middle child of Doris and Harry Feinberg. She has an older brother, Larry, and a younger brother, Art. Harry was a strikingly handsome and charming man who worked in linen sales. Larry is a brilliant and scholarly graduate of St. John's College who has a passion for the arts, classical philosophy, opera, and ballet, which he enjoys in New York City as much as he can. Doris adored Larry, and if she did not have his intellectual heft, she shared his passions.

Art is a very charming guy and something of a comedian, at least to his sister Fern, whom he keeps in stitches. His two mathematically gifted kids, Maggie and Jessie, went on to become engineers, and Art has had a good career as a school psychologist. This was by no means ensured, as Art was initially not much of a student and in the 1960s could easily have lost his way. Fiercely protective, Doris did what was needed to get Art back in the direction of the good life he enjoyed.

During the summers in later years Fern and I would bring our kids, Dan and Jessica, to visit their grandparents.

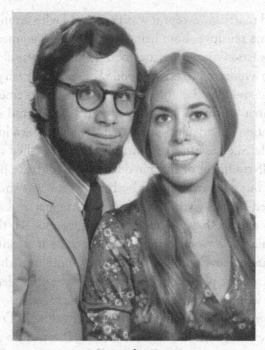

Engaged to Fern

I remember many a pleasant eve sipping good scotch with Harry, Art, and Larry, getting pleasantly mellow with Dan and Jessica underfoot.

Doris, my mother-in-law, was one of the most naturally kind people I ever knew. She spearheaded a lengthy visit from a South African child who stayed with the Feinbergs for many weeks while receiving medical treatment in Philadelphia. Doris was hardly a conventional "Jewish mother," and Fern sometimes bemoaned the fact that she did not get much guidance from her. Doris's style was more to lead by example. She was a patron of the arts in support of Philadelphia's Barnes Foundation, she loved and quoted William Shakespeare, and she loved the outdoors, making sure that after family dinners we went for long walks along Wissahickon Creek.

Doris abhorred and avoided the competitiveness of more conventional Jewish social circles, but she had many loyal friends who loved her. She had brothers and one younger sister, Pauline, with whom she was extremely close. Pauline had a daughter, Fran, who was born within a month of Fern, and they grew up together almost like sisters. Alan, Pauline's son, served in Vietnam as a medic. PBS later produced a documentary on the medics of the Vietnam War, in which he was featured.

Doris and Harry were married for over sixty years. They clearly loved each other, and though they were never rich, they enjoyed every drop of life they could.

In May 1971 I proposed to Fern at the Café Polonaise, a cute little joint near my apartment on Connecticut Avenue. Thankfully, she accepted. The next night when I came to pick her up her at her apartment, her three roommates were all

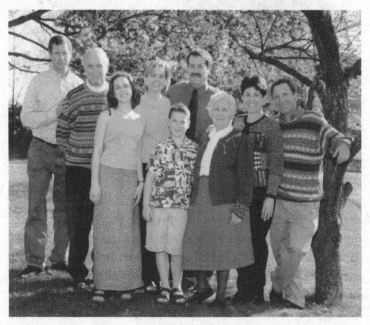

Doris and Harry's Sixtieth Anniversary

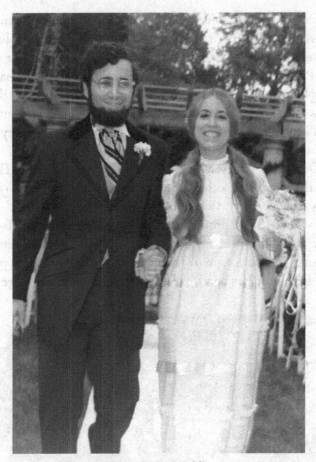

Happy Hippy Wedding

over me, smothering me with hugs and kisses. I hadn't known that they liked me that much. Or maybe they were just looking forward to the extra bedroom. We got married in October in a beautiful spot called Curtis Arboretum, coincidentally the same place I'd had a bar mitzvah party thirteen and a half years before. Our album shows a bunch of hirsute hippies having a great time.

It was a very good year.

Institute of the
Pennsylvania Hospital

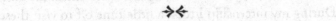

The Residency Years

AS A FOURTH-YEAR MED STUDENT at Penn Med, having chosen psychiatry as my specialty, I was not sure which were the best programs in other parts of the country. The two best in Philadelphia were the residencies at the University of Pennsylvania—excellent but geared for individuals inclined to research and academic psychiatry—and the Institute of the Pennsylvania Hospital, which was affiliated with the Pennsylvania Hospital, the oldest hospital in the country. The institute was our country's oldest psychiatric hospital, and its history was bound to the history of psychiatric care in the United States since before the time of the American Revolution.

The Institute of the Pennsylvania Hospital of 1970 was by far the most prestigious hospital and residency in the Philadelphia area. The best psychiatrists and psychoanalysts trained there. I had enjoyed my learning experiences at the institute in my basic psychiatry rotation, under the tutelage of Dr. Newell Fischer, and during my first fourth-year elective, a two-month stint on the Adolescent Unit, directed by Dr. Lawrence Applebaum, where I fell in love with psychiatry. More about him later.

Given my familiarity with the institute and its familiarity with me, I was very inclined to apply and hopefully go there, but I wanted to at least visit a few programs in other parts of the country. The medical student director, George Ruff, suggested that I apply to the University of Chicago, Johns Hopkins University, the Massachusetts Mental Health Center in Boston, and the University of Rochester, where the psychiatry program was then headed by Jon Romano, a giant in the field at the time.

During my internship I took a little time off to visit these programs.

Rochester was very good and very biologically oriented. The residents were required to wear white coats, which for some reason turned me off. I guess I'd had enough of "whites" as an intern. It is now standard practice, as it should be. One of my interviewers was a very nice psychiatrist who, among other things, asked me why I wasn't married. (Was it supposed to be a measure of emotional stability?) Fern and I were not engaged yet, and I defensively answered that I did have a girlfriend. At the end of the day, they were kind enough to offer me a place.

The University of Chicago was by far the best program I visited, including the Institute of the Pennsylvania Hospital. Aside from the tremendous variety of clinical experiences available and a top-notch faculty, the University of Chicago had a really distinguished psychoanalytic facility. The chairman of the department was Dr. Daniel Freedman, coauthor of the definitive psychiatric textbook of the day, and he interviewed me briefly. Unfortunately, I stayed in a hotel in downtown Chicago and took an elevated train to South Chicago, where the university was, riding over miles and miles of some of the most burned-out slums I'd ever seen. It looked like a war zone. The hospitals were situated in this environment. Despite the superiority of the program, I wasn't sure about living there for three years.

Johns Hopkins was a short drive from DC. Today it is one of the two or three best programs in the country, but then it was poorly organized and was staffed by mostly part-time faculty. I was told that I'd have plenty of time to "teach myself." I suppose that the main selling point would have been being able to hang a Johns Hopkins diploma on your office wall. Who would know?

The Massachusetts Mental Health Center was a highly competitive, very psychoanalytically oriented program in Boston. I was interviewed by the infamous Dr. Harris Funkenstein. Legend had it that he would interview prospective Harvard medical students in a deliberately overheated office. About halfway through the interview, the story went, he would complain of the heat and ask the candidate to open the window, which was nailed shut, so he could see how the candidate handled the stress. Funkenstein didn't do that to me, but I recall that my interview was pretty stressful anyway. It didn't matter, as I was turned down.

Some weeks later, I got a phone call from Dr. Freedman offering me a place at the University of Chicago. Obviously, I wasn't their first choice. I guess there were others who didn't like the neighborhood. I thanked him for the offer but had by then committed to the Institute of the Pennsylvania Hospital. I guess the people at the institute remembered me from when I was a med student there, because I didn't need an interview.

Today psychiatry residencies are four years, the first year of which is devoted to internal medicine, neurology, and inpatient psychiatry as well as emergency medicine and emergency psychiatry, which are assigned through a match program. In a match program, med students list their residency choices in order of preference and residencies list their candidates in order of preference, and the highest choices for each are matched by a computer and revealed in spring of the fourth year of med school on a day called Match Day. When I started there was no match program, so there were separate interviews and selection for internship and residency.

The Institute of the Pennsylvania Hospital, located at Forty-Ninth and Market Streets, was the private psychiatric facility associated with Pennsylvania Hospital, a teaching hospital for the University of Pennsylvania located at Eighth and Spruce Streets. The institute consisted of two parts. The Center Building looked like an old somewhat shabby Main Line hotel, with aging but expensive rugs and furnishings. (Philadelphians refer to Lancaster Avenue as it passes through some of the oldest and wealthiest towns in the suburbs as the Main Line). This was a place where wealthy alcoholic Main Liners went to dry out or where rich people deposited their crazy old uncles. It also contained the offices of a number of prominent psychiatrists.

The North Building was where most of our training took place. Much more modern in appearance, it housed the Inpatient Unit, the Adolescent Unit, residents' and attendings' offices, seminar rooms, and administrative offices.

June 30, 1971, was the last day I wore whites in my career, traded on July 1, 1971, for the sports jacket and tie of the first-year psychiatry resident.

There were five of us in my initial residency group; we were joined by two more after they had completed six months of medical internship at Eighth Street. We were a bright and enthusiastic group, mostly graduates of medical schools in the Philadelphia area: Penn, Jefferson, Temple, and Hahnemann. The teaching faculty was small but consisted of outstanding teachers and role models for the most part. They were very well dressed and very much looked the part of the "Institute psychiatrist," very Brooks Brothers (actually Jacob Reed, this being Philadelphia).

I won't mention all of them, just some who had the most pronounced influence on my professional development.

Newell Fischer was in charge of medical student education, so I first got to know him as a third-year med student. He was a brilliant psychoanalyst and teacher who later became president of the American Psychoanalytic Association. He was puckish and affable, sported a small goatee, and was married to a child psychiatrist. He was one of the first who encouraged my interest in psychiatry. His grasp of the inner working of the minds of our patients was phenomenal.

Myer Mendelson was a wonderful teacher and scholar. Short and bald with large ears, he was soft-spoken and a little self-effacing. But he was definitely not a Brooks Brothers type, and he sometimes had spots on his tie, but his intellectual brilliance and clarity of thought were undeniable. He was not a psychoanalyst, which diminished his stature among the psychoanalyst-laden faculty, but was in fact a world expert on psychoanalytic theories of depression and had written a number of books on the subject.

At one of our weekly conferences, Mendelson presented a man who was chronically depressed. The patient was a professor of philosophy at nearby Swarthmore College, and his specialty was existentialist philosophy, a perfect choice given his persistent frame of mind. He had been fully psychoanalyzed not once but twice by two of the most distinguished psychoanalysts in the Philadelphia area. Here was a man with the deepest level of self-knowledge times two, but he was still miserable when he sought Dr. Mendelson's care.

Dr. Mendelson placed him on desipramine, one of the new tricyclic antidepressants. The patient reported that within a few weeks he was feeling "better than I had in my entire life." He was more productive professionally, and he was able to enjoy his wife and family as he never had before. The effect persisted for months, up to and including the time of the conference. The psychoanalysts were not impressed. This was a "medical cure," a "flight into health" (a defense mechanism in psychoanalytic parlance in which the patient feels consciously better but is actually repressing his still unresolved neurosis). But I was impressed. In fact, I was blown away by the fact that medication had so quickly produced changes that the standard of care of the day, psychoanalytic treatment, had utterly failed to bring about. As far as I was concerned, this alteration in the man's brain chemistry effected a real and more or less permanent change in his mental state.

Many of the other doctors called Mendelson "Myer Medicine" behind his back. But he was the first to stimulate my lifelong interest in biological psychiatry. He was a sweet man, a kind of absentminded professor in appearance, and years later I named my beagle after him.

As first-year residents, we were mostly involved with inpatient psychiatry. We were pretty pampered, and we purposely weren't assigned a large caseload. We were given patients who, it was felt, were good teaching cases under varying degrees of supervision by the attendings. We treated acutely ill patients, mostly schizophrenic, manic-depressives, psychotic individuals with a variety of diagnoses and severe depressives. We developed basic skills in their management with antipsychotics, antidepressants, antianxiety agents, lithium, electroconvulsive therapy (ECT), and various psychotherapeutic modalities. We were only on call weekly, when we stayed in the hospital and took care of the psychiatric and medical needs of all North and Center Building patients. If there was a medical emergency, we would do what we could until transferring the patient by ambulance to the general hospital at Eighth Street.

Once, Dr. Mendelson had an inpatient whom he presented, a beautiful young woman who was admitted to the hospital for "acting bizarrely." When she was presented in morning rounds, she was totally composed and gorgeous. Her husband was there, a portly worried-looking accountant in a three-piece suit.

The history was that the patient and her husband had recently married and were apparently happily. A few months later, she began to take an interest in some kind of consciousness-raising seminar given by a local guru named Peter. These things were pretty common in the early 1970s. She began to attend more and more of his lectures, some of which lasted quite late. Eventually, she informed her husband that she was in love with her guru and intended to move in with him, along with some of his other acolytes. At the same time, she was acting oddly at home and staying up all night. The husband felt that she was acting strangely and had her admitted to the institute.

She presented as very coherent that morning after taking something for sleep. She did not show pressured speech or bizarre thought process and explained matter-of-factly that she was no longer in love with her husband. Her mind, she said, had been expanded by her guru, and she intended for her life to go in another direction. Fueled by our little crushes on her and full of contempt for her frantic, straitlaced accountant husband, we residents completely bought into this. We simply could not understand why Dr. Mendelson was going along with hospitalizing a person for a "lifestyle change."

Dr. Mendelson insisted that she was manic and psychotic, just presenting in a more subtle fashion than we were used to. He put her on lithium carbonate.

The patient figured that she wouldn't get back to her guru if she didn't go along with the program, and she took her lithium as directed.

About a week later, she was presented again in morning rounds. She looked somehow different and stated, "I don't understand what got into me. My husband has been so loving and patient while I was acting like an idiot. What could I have seen in that ridiculous Peter?" She then tearfully asked for her husband's forgiveness, which he gladly gave. The husband turned to Dr. Mendelson and said, "Thank you for giving me my wife back."

Sometime later Joseph, a young man who had been a high school classmate of mine, was admitted to the hospital. I remembered him being something of a snob who wouldn't give me the time of day. His presentation, however, was the opposite of subtle, a severe hypermanic state with manic excitement, sleeplessness, nongoal-directed hyperactivity, and incoherent rambling, a state that if untreated can end in death.

His attending, a pompous windbag named Jerry Gottenberg, admitted Joseph to the psychiatric intensive care unit, which was essentially an isolation unit. Dr. Gottenberg treated him with hypnotics (sleeping medication), allowing Joseph to get some sleep, while visiting him daily for weeks, offering him psychoanalytic interpretations of his psychotic state, which did not improve. Gottenberg's resident, a very bright and savvy guy named Harvey Horowitz, begged Gottenberg to start Joseph on lithium, which after a few weeks he reluctantly agreed to do.

Sure enough, within a week Joseph de-escalated to an essentially euthymic (normal mood) state. Don't ask me how many brain cells were destroyed while he went untreated. I would chat with him as he came to recognize me, and we reminisced a bit about Central High School. I was glad that he was better, but I admit to being a little pleased that I was the resident and that the snob was the mental patient.

There was an attending, a research psychiatrist named Martin Orne, a world expert on hypnosis who had devoted his life to research on the subject. He was internationally famous, wrote many books and articles, and founded the American Society of Clinical Hypnosis and edited its journal. He traveled all over the country to testify in criminal trials about the use of hypnosis in the legal process. Dr. Orne gave a course in hypnosis techniques and practice that was open to senior residents as well as physicians and dentists in the Philadelphia area. The course was popular and usually oversubscribed. I took it and became skilled in the techniques he taught and used them in my work for years to come.

Dr. Orne also gave a seminar on scientific and statistical methods in psychiatry, and we were taught how to read scientific literature critically and analyze the quality of research. Science is at heart a method and attitude that can be applied to any inquiry well or badly. In his clear and intellectually rigorous thought and sonorous voice, Dr. Orne was able to impart what all this meant. I was a medical student and a chemistry major in college, but I really only came to appreciate how science was done because of Orne's seminar.

As part of the course requirements, we each had to design a protocol on a topic of our choice. Dr. Orne told me that my protocol was as good as what he'd seen from the best of his PhD students, and he encouraged me to make research a part of my career. It was one of the greatest compliments I have ever received, but I knew myself well enough to know that I really lacked the energy and driving curiosity necessary to be a good researcher. I was meant to be a clinician.

Second-year residency was devoted to halftime outpatient psychiatry and six months of consultation psychiatry at Pennsylvania Hospital and six months at the inpatient Adolescent Unit. Outpatient cases were mostly psychoanalytically oriented psychotherapy, and we had for the most part very smart psychoanalytically trained supervisors. We also followed a few of the sicker patients we had treated as inpatients the previous year. I enjoyed monitoring and treating with medications those chronically seriously ill patients.

I learned a lot about therapeutic restraint and neutrality as well as the ability to spot transference on the part of patients and to manage my own countertransference, the feelings that therapists naturally develop toward their patients. Technically these feelings arise from the therapist's own past relationships, but they're generally experienced and understood as feelings toward the patient. You try to use those feelings in the patient's best interests, partly by not acting on them inappropriately. I think that all physicians should be better trained in this, though I think I had a natural ability to handle those feelings.

We were also on call for ER psychiatry every two weeks and were in charge of the treatment and disposition of psychiatric emergencies at Eighth Street, presenting cases to the attending the following morning.

The Adolescent Unit was populated by a combination of severely mentally ill adolescents with schizophrenia, manic depression, anorexia nervosa, and other maladies, along with substance abusers. The substance abusers were mostly heroin addicts who tended to be the incorrigible offspring of wealthy people from all over the United States; they often remained at the institute for months or until Daddy's money ran out.

I was entranced by my experience on the unit as a med student. It sealed my choice of psychiatry as a specialty. I developed a more realistic view as a resident.

The director, Dr. Larry Applebaum, was a charismatic man who was arrogant, self-assured, and somewhat narcissistic. He trusted his gut more than anything and was, I suspected, an admirer of antipsychiatrists such as Thomas Szasz.

I couldn't stand the guy, but he was the greatest natural psychotherapist I've ever known. I wanted to be able to do psychotherapy with his exuberant flair.

Every morning, there would be a meeting on the unit led by Applebaum and one of the residents. This was in fact a large group therapy session that included patients, residents, therapists, and teachers (there was a high school at the institute).

Dr. Applebaum seemed to have a complete grasp of the group's dynamics and of what was going on in the heads of the various psychotics, psychopaths, and drug addicts and how they related in a group setting to each other and the rest of us. The morning meeting was his chance to do psychotherapy as performance art. His interpretations of what was going on sometimes went over my head, but he was able to help the kids therapeutically with their intense and sometimes out-of-control feelings about themselves and others and did so remarkably well. I hope that some of him soaked into me. One can be taught to do competent psychotherapy, but the great ones have a natural talent too. It requires an enormous amount of empathy and the ability to know how and when to communicate to patients in a therapeutic manner. Charisma helps too, and Applebaum had a lot of it.

As residents we were able to do group family and marital therapy, and we were trained by experts in the various treatments. Third-year residency was essentially an outpatient year, with plenty of time for electives. I was grateful that even though the institute was psychoanalytically oriented, it allowed me to pursue my interests without interference. If the institute didn't offer something, I was able to go outside the program to find it, which mostly was at the University of Pennsylvania.

The residents were also encouraged to begin a personal psychoanalysis in preparation for psychoanalytic training. Ten years before if you were a smart and ambitious resident, you would invariably become a psychoanalyst. I don't think any of our group did. Today psychoanalysis has been sidelined in favor of shorter-term more evidence-based therapies, such as cognitive behavioral and dialectic behavioral therapies, which have dependably proven to be successful. Psychopharmacology is catching up to other pharmacologies in medicine, with genetics and neuroscience pointing the way to more scientifically targeted therapies. More subtle forms of ECT, transcranial-magnet therapies, deep-brain stimulation, and even carefully mapped neurosurgical procedures for intractable psychiatric conditions round out modern choices for psychiatrists and their patients.

Once in one of our first-year conferences, a manic-depressive inpatient was presented by a guest at the institute who was a world expert on the psychoanalytic interpretation and treatment of manic depression. One of the residents asked him what he thought of lithium's place in treatment (a medication that had by then been available for a number of years). The world expert admitted that he didn't know much about lithium.

About a year later I attended a conference at one of the psychoanalytic academies in Philadelphia. I don't recall the precise topic, but one of the discussants was Emanuel Peterfreund, a classically trained analyst from New York City who was a professor at one of the medical schools there. He also was a brilliant and original thinker who had done a lot of work using computer-based models of the mind, ideas that were original for the early 1970s. I found his ideas dazzling, and I thought that even if you disagreed with him, his ideas clearly deserved to be considered and discussed.

The others on the panel apparently disagreed with my opinion. They couldn't wait to express their barely concealed contempt for an apostate who dared to question or reinterpret the Freudian model and mechanisms of how the mind worked, and they responded with uniformly vituperative dismissals of his views. The head of the conference must have been embarrassed by how a colleague, even one who strayed from orthodoxy, was being treated. Even his remarks were patronizing.

Peterfreund was a heretic and not to be tolerated. I remember thinking that if I wanted a career in religion I'd have become a rabbi. So much for becoming a psychoanalyst.

The work of Masters and Johnson was gaining prominence at that time, and I took training in the treatment of sexual dysfunction at the Marriage Counsel, which was a part of the University of Pennsylvania. This too became part of my tool kit. Behavioral therapy, the predecessor to the cognitive-behavioral therapy practiced today, was pioneered by two Philadelphia psychiatrists, Joseph Wolpe of Temple and Aaron Beck at Penn. I was interested in behavioral therapy and took a supervisor from Penn to train with. I learned many techniques and misapplied them.

The patient I misapplied them to was Bob, a likable engineering grad student from Penn who grew up in a working-class family in western Pennsylvania. His complaint was essentially "I'm homosexual and I don't want to be." I took a thorough history. Bob had been attracted to boys and men for as long as he could remember and, due to a number of factors, despised the fact and wanted to change. He hated being gay, and his father, a gruff steelworker, would rather have his son dead than accept him as gay.

Bob had no effeminate mannerisms, so his sexual preference was not externally apparent. He was reasonably good-looking and dated many women. On occasion he experienced heterosexual sex, but it did nothing much for him. In grad school, he'd secretly been leading a gay life.

Even at the start I doubted that any therapy would change his orientation, and I tried to persuade him that it almost certainly wouldn't work. But he wanted to try, and for my part, I wanted to practice all these wonderful skills I was learning.

We used operant and aversive conditioning and hypnotic imagery, mixed in with more traditional psychotherapy. At first things seemed encouraging. He found himself a girlfriend and was sexually active with her. He even brought her in for sexual counseling, and she was fully aware of what we were doing. He liked her and she was in love with him, but it just wasn't working.

At one point I asked Bob if he liked porn films. He said that he watched them and was always turned on by the guy. I then had a "brilliant" idea. I went to the Marriage Counsel, which had a fully stocked film library of educational films. I asked the librarian if there were any films in the library for lesbians with sex problems. Her acerbic response was to ask me if I was a lesbian with a sex problem. I drew myself up and huffed that I was a senior resident at the institute. I had a patient who needed help, and I believed that this could be a way to help him. After signing my life away in triplicate, I rushed back to my office to view what were basically lesbian sex films.

They couldn't be less like the typical, seedy, badly filmed black-and-white porn flicks of the day. The sex was in incredible, erotic, living color, and the women in the films—actresses? therapists?—were gorgeous. Technically I guess they were considered sex therapists, but that seemed to be stretching the definition a bit.

My bright idea was that Bob might be aroused by watching beautiful lesbians go at it, and while I could barely contain my arousal the first time I showed the films in one of his therapy sessions, Bob could barely stay awake.

That was not the end of it, though. One of the other residents had noticed that I was using a projector in my office and asked me what I had been using it for. I said that it was an educational film, but I couldn't say any more. "Confidentiality, you know."

"C'mon Hoffman. If it's a treatment technique, shouldn't you share with your fellow residents?"

I fessed up.

A few nights later, my office was the location of what might have been the most fully and enthusiastically attended clinical conference in the history of the institute.

After the "conference" I was, at least to my fellow residents, the hero of the moment. "Hoffman, you are a true scholar, and that was clearly our finest educational experience to date, a real teaching moment. Can we do this every week?"

Unfortunately, Bob did not benefit a bit. I hope that he wasn't too embarrassed sitting through all of those films.

I hope that in the end, I was able to help him better accept who he was. As for me, I learned about limitations of treatment. I did get to write up a case study on Bob, which was a requirement to complete residency.

I'm sorry to say that the Institute of the Pennsylvania Hospital closed its doors permanently in 1997. It failed financially, perhaps because it didn't change enough with the times. The Massachusetts General Hospital in Boston and McLean Hospital, institutions comparable to the University of Pennsylvania and the Institute of the Pennsylvania Hospital, successfully combined their programs to become what is arguably the best program in the country. I have often thought that in combination, the best of Penn and the best of the institute may have been the same.

I think I put that program together for myself when I was there.

Boards

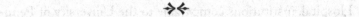

SHORTLY AFTER THE END of residency, I began the grueling process of preparing for and taking psychiatry boards. Passing meant "proof" of competence in your specialty and was given yearly by the American Board of Psychiatry and Neurology. The written exam, which was one-third neurology and two-thirds psychiatry, was comprehensive in testing knowledge of adult and child psychiatry, schizophrenia, bipolar disorders, depression, anxiety, OCD, ADD, personality disorders, psychopharmacology, toxic interactions among all drugs (psychiatric or not), psychoanalytic theory, behavioral and analytically oriented therapies, group and family therapies, and substantial parts of neurology, particularly those relevant to psychiatric practice such as the dementias, parkinsonism, and multiple sclerosis.

The second part, the orals, taken after passing the written exam, were given two years later and were much scarier. They were administered in a distant city (in my case Los Angeles). The orals consisted of three one-hour exams, one in neurology and two in psychiatry, one half hour of which was to be spent taking the histories of three actual patients followed by a neurological exam or the mental status exam.

My first oral exam took place in a small spare conference room with white walls, little decoration, and a plain conference table behind which sat two rather unsympathetic-looking examiners. They perfunctorily introduced themselves to me. Heart pounding, I felt like I was in Sartre's "No Exit" waiting room. Then the patient was invited in.

There was a rumor that anyone who didn't start by introducing himself and thanking the patient for coming would be immediately failed for "not establishing rapport." I did not test its truthfulness.

I recall that one of the psychiatric patients was actively psychotic and experiencing auditory hallucinations. When this happens especially in an initial evaluation, you must ask if the voices are telling the patient to harm himself or others, which I fortunately remembered to do (not do, not pass!).

After observing your technique, the examiner asked you to discuss your findings and possible diagnoses and include any further studies that you felt would be helpful. In the psychiatric assessment you were expected give a formulation of the patient's psychopathology and a specific treatment plan, including medications and type of psychotherapy indicated.

In the neurology oral you were instructed to interpret the abnormalities of your neurological exam, including what parts of the brain, the spinal column, or peripheral nerves were functioning abnormally and what diseases might cause this. The psychiatrists, I'm sure, were cut a little slack here, as were the neurologists for the psych oral.

After eight nerve-racking weeks I received a telegram thankfully stating that I had passed. I got an impressive-looking certificate, which I framed and hung in my office. This proved that on a particular date on a particular year I knew enough psychiatry and neurology to pass a comprehensive examination and two years later had enough control over my anxiety to do a straightforward evaluation successfully.

In those days, once you were board certified it was forever. Continuing education was on the honor system (though required for keeping state medical licenses).

Subsequently, all specialists have had to to recertify at least every ten years with various maintenance of certification requirements in between. This has become a cottage industry for review course givers and review book writers.

Most doctors don't have to be told to keep up in their fields. For me, taking yearly courses in psychiatry, psychopharmacology, and from time to time neurology, neuroscience, and internal medicine is always interesting and a good excuse to take minivacations to New York, Boston, Chicago, Vail, Killington in Vermont, or . . . you get the idea.

My First Day
in the Air Force

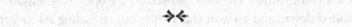

AFTER THREE LONG DAYS of driving, Fern and I finally arrived in Biloxi, Mississippi, where, at Keesler Air Force Base Medical Center I was to begin my brief career as a US Air Force psychiatrist. It was the 1970s, just at the end of the Vietnam War era.

I was a Berry Planner. The Berry Plan was a method of drafting doctor "volunteers" during the Vietnam War. If the military needed certain specialties, it would grant deferments year to year during residency training. In your senior year in medical school, you joined a particular branch of the military and were a reserve officer during your internship and residency. The training director provided yearly letters to your draft board certifying that you had successfully completed the training year. Otherwise, bingo! You got to go to Vietnam as a general medical officer. Ironically, I had a high draft number, which means that if I hadn't been a doctor I would not have had to enter military service at all.

In my year, the air force apparently decided that it was a waste of military resources to send Berry Planners to basic training. It was the only year in air force history that there were midrank military officers who had not received one instant of basic training. That lack of basic training sometimes became obvious.

Several months later I was walking on base with a few colleagues, including Major Al Gardner, a great guy and a really good psychiatrist but the least military among us. He was walking along with his shirttail hanging out, flapping in the breeze. Down the main drag heading toward us came a large black limo with a little flag bearing two stars on each bumper, indicating that the passenger was Major General Schotts, the base commander. The limo slowed to a stop, a rear window rolled down, and an arm was thrust out, signaling Al to "get over here." Al walked over with a "What did I do?" look on his face. The arm pointed to the shirttail, which Al sheepishly tucked. We were watching and cringing, certain that poor Al was about to get the dressing down of his life if not a court-martial. But all Schotts said was "Now get out of my sight."

The following year, basic training was reinstated.

After spending a long day in various lines, being issued uniforms and ID badges and filling out endless forms, Fern and I finally got to go home to the three-bedroom house assigned to us on base, entirely excessive for a couple with no children but apparently the mandatory size for a major, and we moved in immediately.

Early that first evening, Fern made an innocent request.

"Jeff, why don't you drive onto the base, get some gas, and stop at the commissary to pick up a few groceries while I check out the house?"

"Okay. How hard can that be?"

After gassing up our aging but reliable 1970 Duster, now festooned with a blue bumper sticker indicating that it was the car of an officer, I made off for the commissary, doing roughly eighteen miles per hour in a fifteen-mile-per-hour zone.

Within seconds lights were flashing behind me, and I pulled the car to the side of the road. Two airmen in white helmets approached my car, saluted smartly, and politely asked me for my driver's license, registration, and military ID.

"Sir, you were exceeding the speed limit in a fifteen-mile-per-hour zone."

I was later to learn that speed limits are taken very literally on a military base. The military police officers looked at my papers and seemed to spend an inordinate amount of time examining both sides of my military ID, which identified me as Major Jeffrey Hoffman, USAF.

After what seemed forever, the policemen returned to the car, once again saluting, then "asking" me, "Sir, would you please follow our Jeep."

"What have I done now?" I wondered as I followed the Jeep to the Keesler Air Force Base police station.

I was directed to a seat in front of the desk sergeant and was again asked for my ID. "Sergeant," I boldly asked, "I know I was speeding, but don't they just give tickets in the air force?"

The sergeant looked at me suspiciously and said, "Your ID says Major Jeffrey Hoffman."

"That's right. I'm in the medical corps. I just got here."

"Your ID doesn't have a medical corps stamp on the other side."

"Is it supposed to?" I asked innocently.

I was at this moment in time twenty-nine years old and thin, and with my ultrashort military haircut I looked ten years younger, pretty much like your average recruit who came to Keesler for schooling after basic training. In other words, I was being detained for impersonating an officer.

The sergeant wasn't quite sure what to make of my story but asked me who my immediate commanding officer was. "Um, that would be Lieutenant Colonel Paul Kantack," who was then chairman of the psychiatry department and an air force lifer whom I had yet to meet, as actual hospital duty was not to start until the next day. The sergeant said that he would try to contact Kantack at home.

Fortunately, the sergeant was able to reach Kantack. Unfortunately, Kantack had no idea who I was, but he was kind enough to search through his list of new staff officers and was finally able to identify me. I imagine the colonel must have thought to himself "I haven't even met this asshole, and he managed to get himself arrested."

As I left the police station, the sergeant snickered and advised me "Sir, be sure to get your medical corps stamp on your ID ASAP."

I arrived home about two hours after leaving for a quick grocery run, and my wife was angry and relieved at the same time.

"What the hell happened to you? I thought maybe they shipped you to Vietnam."

"Fern you'll never believe this, but ..."

Day Two and Beyond,
US Air Force

My second official active-duty day was my first day of actually wearing the US Air Force uniform. It was also the day I was introduced to my duties and the department chairman, Lieutenant Colonel Paul Kantack, who already knew my name from my "arrest" the day before.

Kantack was an air force lifer who was perhaps five years older than me. It seemed as if he was really trying to play the role of a hard-ass but was just a bit too goofy for the part. We grew to like him. We called him "Boss," and he pretty much let us be psychiatrists, caring for our patients with as little interference as possible. My new colleagues were all Berry Planners, one of whom was a med school classmate, a Princetonian I didn't much care for when we were at Penn Med, but Fern and I became very fond of him and his wife during the air force years. All of us were from and had trained in the Northeast, and we were unjustifiably arrogant in Biloxi among military types.

The department also had a number of psychologists, social workers, and enlisted men, many of whom were career air force and served various functions in the department as mental health techs, or psych techs. For the most part we had pretty good camaraderie.

My first assignment was to the inpatient unit, which had a large unlocked section and a smaller locked unit. While the

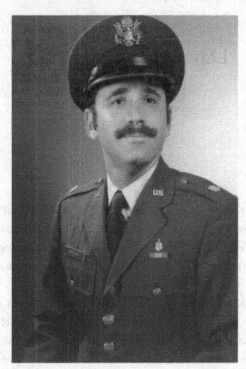

Majorissimo Jeff

department served active-duty members, their families, and retirees, the inpatient unit tended to be populated by acutely ill active-duty air force personnel. Unlike in civilian life, the emergency psychiatrist on call, entirely at his own discretion, could order an active-duty member of any rank onto the inpatient unit. Fortunately, I never had to involuntarily commit a general.

On my first day on the unit, one of the techs approached me gingerly, stating "Uh, sir? I think we have a problem."

"What's that, Sergeant?"

"We, uh, that is, you have a patient, Sergeant Baker, very angry, aggressive, paranoid, and psychotic, over on the locked unit."

"So, I'll see him in a minute. What's the problem?"

"He thinks he's getting discharged—today."

"Who told him that, Sergeant?"

"I think it was Dr. Bond." That was the name of the Berry Planner I was replacing. "Last week, he told Sergeant Baker he should be out in a few days, but he's still hallucinating and pretty psychotic, and you're gonna have to tell your patient his discharge is a little delayed."

Was this a test for the new guy? A trial? A hazing ritual? I was determined to show my courage, not to mention my polished clinical skills. "Okay. Where is he?"

A locked door with a midsize window led to the unit, where Baker, the only current patient, resided along with a large male nurse and no restraints. Even from a distance, Baker looked big, and he looked angry.

"Uh, maybe it would be good if you two came in with me, just for backup."

"Good idea, Doc."

We opened the door, and trying to look confident, I approached Baker. He was a huge African American, at least 250 pounds of solid, muscled rage. The techs didn't follow.

"Good morning. I'm Dr. Hoffman, your new doctor."

No answer, plenty of glare.

"How are you feeling today?"

Threatening glare. "Ready to go home."

"Uh, we need to talk about that."

"Dr. Bond said I could go home today."

"Well, I think we need to delay that a few days you see—"

Suddenly the missile of muscle is lunging toward me, my fight-or-flight reflex in full-flight mode as I rush to the door. But where was my backup?

The psych techs were nowhere to be seen. I shook the door, I was locked in, the psych techs laughing hysterically from the outside.

The nurse held Baker for just a split second while the techs opened the door to let me out, and then the muscle missile was banging his fists from the other side.

"Nice job, Doc." the tech said through tears of laughter.

"You knew this would happen, didn't you?"

"Not exactly, but somebody had to tell him."

I walked away muttering something about whether these two assholes were the best the air force could do for mental health.

Mostly in our outpatient department, where I was eventually made chief, the air force gave me the opportunity to hone skills that I learned as a resident.

One of those skills was medical hypnosis, which has many applications in both psychiatry and general medicine. I started seeing a young recruit named Johnny who was newly married to Louise, whom he called Lou. Lou and Johnny were having serious marital problems, specifically sexual problems. They had been raised in religious-fundamentalist Alabama, and though they apparently loved each other, Lou was repressed, fearful, and guilty, and Johnny had no idea what to do. Possibly affected by many childhood fire-and-brimstone sermons about the wages of sin, their marriage remained unconsummated.

However, every now and then, Lou would find herself waking up in some strange man's bed. Mortified and claiming to have absolutely no recollection of how she got there, she would call Johnny to pick her up. Amazingly, he always did, forgiving her and accepting that she wasn't responsible; it was a demon that had gotten into her and led her there.

I suspected that this could be a case of multiple personality disorder, in which an unacceptably wanton sexual side of Lou was being enacted unconsciously.

Lou turned out to be an excellent hypnotic subject, and it was fairly easy to access her hypersexual alter ego, whom she called "Weesa." Weesa would go to a bar during the day in her fugue state and basically couple with whoever for some uninhibited but dangerous sex. Weesa had apparently come to be before they were married and had contempt for her husband's inexperience, but she admitted that she "kind of loved the guy, anyway."

The treatment process eventually involved introducing the repressed Lou to the uninhibited Weesa in the hypnotic state. The one thing they had in common was that they both cared for the ultraforgiving Johnny. The idea now was to integrate the prim but loyal and loving church girl with the sexually experienced and uninhibited Weesa. I came up with the idea that both her names were childish, and it might help if she referred to herself as Louise.

Believe it or not, as far as I know, Johnny and Louise did well after that. Too good to be true? Maybe, but that's how I remember it.

Penis Envy and Other
Air Force Stories

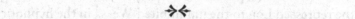

ONE OF OUR FELLOW department members was Nancy, a psychologist and captain whose husband was a captain in the Judge Advocate General's Corps. Nancy was very bright, intense, conscientious, and opinionated. She was cute in a skinny-chicken kind of way. She was definitely not a lifer. Did I mention that she was a feminist?

Every week, one us would present a case or a lecture on a topic of our choosing of general interest to the department. One week, Dr. Al Gardner was to give a lecture titled "Basic Psychoanalytic Concepts." In the mid-1970s psychoanalytic and Freudian theory held great if somewhat waning sway over psychiatry, and a lecture on psychoanalytic ideas was seemingly noncontroversial.

Al took us through the unconscious mind, id, ego, and superego; treatment basics on transference, countertransference, and resistance; and stages of child development, oral, anal, and oedipal. Then came Freud's idea about female psychosexual stages, including penis envy, the unproven and now completely discredited idea that all little girls have an unconscious desire to possess daddy's penis, which is only fully resolved with pregnancy and the birth of a first male child.

> Al: "In Freud's view, penis envy is an unconscious aspect of female psychosexual—"

Nancy (shrieking): "Penis envy!"

Al: "Nancy, you have a question?"

Nancy (reddening): "There's no such thing as penis envy!"

Al: "I'm not advocating it, but it is of basic Freudian—"

Nancy: "I will not sit here and listen to a lecture on penis envy."

Al: "But we can discuss it; refute it if you want."

Nancy: "Another word about penis envy and I'm out of here."

Dr. Kantack: [Stunned silence.]

Al: "Okay, no more penis envy."

Nancy: "That's it!"

Exit Nancy, storming out.

With the lecture ending early that day, Al and I tried to figure out what happened. We concluded that Nancy had a bad case of unresolved you-know-what.

On one occasion my grandfather, age eighty-five, called me up with the idea that he would like to fly down to Biloxi to visit his grandson in the air force. Zeda was thin, balding, and 5′3″, a feisty widower who spoke with a thick Yiddish accent. He was charming but also something of a blowhard. He doted on me, and I loved him.

As a young man, Zeda had deserted from Czar Nicholas II's army and come to the United States, where he earned enough money to bring over my grandmother and father as well as other family members.

I had no hesitation about welcoming him and introducing him around. The southern ladies who were the secretaries in our department thought that he was adorable, talking about himself and me in his unusual accent. I felt proud to show him off and proud that I was the son and grandson of immigrants and had become a doctor in the US Air Force.

After meeting with various staff members, I took Zeda to meet Kantack.

"Dr. Kantack, this is my grandfather, Jacob Hoffman. Zeda, this is Colonel Kantack. He's my boss."

"Very good to meet you, Mr. Hoffman. Your grandson is a fine doctor."

"Thank you. Pleased to meet you."

"So, Mr. Hoffman, what do you think of your grandson being in the air force?"

For the first time during his visit, I was feeling a little nervous about what might come out of Zeda's mouth, the czar's army deserter, whose son had been seriously wounded in World War II.

To my relief Zeda smiled as he replied, "You have to serve your country."

A significant number of air force personnel at Keesler were Jewish, many of them medical officers. There were enough of us to warrant a base chaplain, Rabbi Gold. The rabbi was a career officer, a lieutenant colonel who was also a bit of a rebel. He celebrated all of the holidays of the Jewish calendar, but from the standpoint of our base, by far the most important event was the annual Seder. At Keesler this was not just a Jewish event but also an important ecumenical celebration to which all base luminaries, up to and including Major General Schotts, the base commander, were invited. Schotts was every inch the scion of an old southern military family whose roots and traditions reached back to the Confederacy, and that year he attended the Seder.

The Seder proceeded along traditional lines, led by Rabbi Gold. He told the story of Jewish slavery and liberation from the pharaoh of Egypt, with all of us, including Schotts, taking turns reading portions of the Haggadah and then singing traditional Seder songs.

At the end, Rabbi Gold asked us all to stand up and join hands as he led us in singing "We Shall Overcome," which was a kind of unofficial anthem of the civil rights movement.

Given what Passover is about, you could say that this is a perfectly appropriate addition to the liturgy, but to a southern general it might as well have been the socialists' "Internationale" or "Deutchland Uber Alles."

Shortly, we had a new rabbi.

Dr. Kantack organized the department into small teams responsible for the care of our inpatients and outpatients, each headed by a psychiatrist and a junior officer. My partner was Captain Jones, a very bright social worker. First thing in the morning, our first job was to make rounds on our hospital patients and then divide up responsibilities for their care. I liked Jones, and we got along well. After a while he stopped showing up, intermittently at first and then not at all. I asked him what was wrong more than once. He invariably apologized, promising that it would never happen again, but the no-shows persisted. I asked the boss what he suggested I do, and he recommended a verbal reminder followed by a formal letter. Once again Jones promised to do better, but there was no change, leaving me to do his job on the ward as well as mine.

Part of my job every six months was to do an Officer Efficiency Report (OER), an evaluation of the officer junior to me, which in this case was Jones. Anything less than stellar was the kiss of death to an officer's career, but what could I do? He didn't show up for his job. I gave him average evaluations.

About a week later I was summoned to the office of the hospital commander, Colonel Amdahl. He was the second most important officer at Keesler and was about to be promoted to general.

"I read your OER on Captain Jones. Why are his ratings so low?"

"Sir, he rarely showed up for rounds, and I gave him several verbal warnings and a written warning."

"Did you know he was spending his mornings with me on a special hospital project?"

"No, I didn't, sir."

"Major, I want you to reconsider and revise your OER's for Jones."

I asked Col. Kantack for advice, but he wasn't helpful. He told me to do what I thought was right.

In the end, I didn't change Jones's OER and effectively ended his military career. Had I any aspiration of staying in the air force, I know that I would have been forced to handle the evaluation differently. It was clear that as long as you wore the uniform, your first obligation was to "the Mission," and the mission was whatever the air force thought it was. The chain of command communicated the mission of the air force. In this case, the colonel was the face of the air force. Knowing that I was leaving to go into private practice obviously influenced my decision.

Jones later approached me and said, "I never thought you'd do it. You ruined my career."

I felt bad, but I think that he ruined his own career.

However, I was young and smug, and if I could do it over again I think I would have changed the damn OER.

The most lasting effect that the air force had on me was my politics. My parents were liberal Democrats, and growing up I was too. But the last Democrat I voted for in a presidential election was George McGovern in 1972.

In the air force I experienced a government-run health care system up close. Though there were many good and dedicated physicians who were career air force, I felt that the system protected and, at times, encouraged mediocrity. More important, it was the system, which was termed "the Mission," that always took priority even over the best interests of individual patients. My experience with Captain Jones was an example of this.

I understand that any large system to some extent exists to perpetuate itself, but the air force left me with the impression that unchecked government is the mother of all perpetuators.

I couldn't wait to go into private practice, where I'd be free to advocate for myself and my patients. How naive I was!

But the air force changed me into a Republican, at least in the sense that my personal experience with a centralized health care system made me suspicious of the efficacy of centralized government systems of all sorts. I do not regret my years in the air force, though. The air force gave me the opportunity to hone my professional skills, enjoy new colleagues and friends, and serve my country all at the same time.

Mendelson

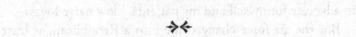

MISSISSIPPI WAS RABBIT-HUNTING COUNTRY, and for rabbits you need rabbit dogs (known everywhere else in the world as beagles). Therefore, Mississippi had world-class beagle breeders. Fern and I had no children at the time, so we decided to adopt a dog. We put a lot of thought into it. "Beagles are cute. There are lots of beagles around here. Let's get one!" we reasoned.

We went to our local beagle farm and found ourselves an adorable, frolicky six-week-old little fellow. Since we had two empty bedrooms we decided to give him his own room, and Fern made him his own little doggie bed in the base wood shop. But the first night the doggie whimpered pitifully, so we took him to our bed, where he quieted down peacefully and we bonded eternally.

A few nights later, we had some of our air force friends over for dinner: Sue and Louie Reich (the Princeton guy), Marie and Al Gardner (flapping shirttail guy), and Nancy (penis envy) and Cap. Potter. Fern made a bunch of meatballs and spaghetti, and we all got pretty drunk on Chianti. I introduced our new little doggie, and Louie asked, "What have you named him?"

"Don't know yet. Maybe you guys can help us out."

After coming up with a bunch of names, some funny, many obscene, and all inappropriate, Al asked, "Does he remind you of anyone?"

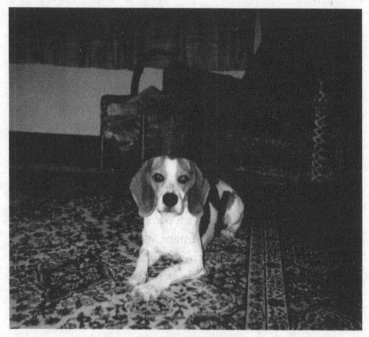

Doggie Mendelson

Doggie had a smooth head, large floppy ears, and an endearing quizzical expression.

"This may sound crazy, but he reminds me of Myer Mendelson," I said, remembering the Penn professor who influenced me so much during residency. Our company insisted, and we agreed. The dog was Mendelson. We eventually sobered up, but we kept the name.

He was, as happens to many, our first son, and we loved him, danced with him, and enjoyed him thoroughly. When Dan and Jessica, our children, came along, Mendelson was a terrific playmate for them, and he endured their mauling dutifully or retreated underneath the couch. Not that Mendelson was perfect. He turned out to be pretty stupid and was often disobedient. So, we took him to air force obedience school, where he got a D minus, the lowest grade ever given. The trainer said that Mendelson would have flunked if he weren't an officer's dog. He shed a lot too.

Mendelson would often run off into the night to do God knows what, and I would chase him through the neighborhood, finally nabbing him blocks away. When we got home he would assume the guilty supplicant posture as I yelled at him, but I could never get really angry at him, and I think he knew it. He was so full of love and unquestioning affection.

Years later when Mendelson got really ill with cancer, we reluctantly euthanized him with the sympathy and help of an understanding vet. The Hoffmans were grief-stricken. I am not a crier, but tears came from a place in me that I hardly knew existed. Fern and the kids were inconsolable too. But we have lots of pictures, and they make us all smile.

Real Life

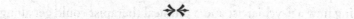

My time in the US Air Force was rapidly drawing to a close, and Fern and I had to figure out where we wanted to live and work. We had a few ideas but nothing really clear. I was willing to consider anywhere, and Fern was okay with being close to family but not necessarily Philadelphia. Even then we both liked the idea of moving to Florida, but getting a medical license there was close to impossible. I looked at jobs in the Washington, DC, area and the Philly and greater Boston areas. There was a very good hospital called Carrier Clinic near Princeton, New Jersey, where one of my fellow residents was on staff. For some reason I was intimidated by the place and the guy who interviewed me, a pompous bow-tied director, and I didn't pursue it any further than that interview.

I had family north of Boston and fond memories of growing up in the area. I had no concept of the practicalities of living in Massachusetts or starting a practice there, but Fern and I decided to go for it. You learn fast. I had no job, no practice, and no professional contacts, nor did I really know if the North Shore of Boston needed psychiatrists. I rented an office in Lynnfield, an upscale suburb of Lynn ("Lynn, Lynn, city of sin"), a small coastal, fading industrial city. I thought that it might be a good location but really had no sure idea. We figured that with our savings, we could afford to live for a year even if nobody came.

The suite was to be shared with a physical therapist, Rich Whalen, who had been there less than a year. Richard was a medic in Vietnam and decided on his career partly because of his war experiences. Fern was my office manager, and Donna, Rich's wife, was his. Donna was a pretty, soft-spoken, unselfish person with whom Fern got along with famously, explaining how a psychiatrist and a physical therapist could get along so well for almost twenty years sharing the same suite.

When Rich and I started working together neither of us had kids, but we subsequently each had a son and a daughter of the same ages, so we were able to share the joys and tribulations of our children over the years. Distance now separates us, but we are still good friends with the Whelans.

I joined the staff of a few local hospitals and let my fingers do the walking through the local yellow pages. I picked at random the names of about fifty local general practitioners, internists, and ob-gyns—the primary-care doctors most likely to refer patients to a psychiatrist—whom I proceeded to cold-call. Surprisingly, about half of them invited me to visit their offices, and of those about a dozen slowly began referring patients to me.

The advice I received as I was starting out was cheap and plentiful, but the only I remember was that "to be a success, have availability, affability, and ability," of which the third was the least important.

Fern and I were living in El Cheapo apartments in Beverly, so the cost of living was manageable, and Fern worked for a while at a place called the Landmark School, which schooled students with learning disabilities. I also took a couple of part-time jobs at nearby mental health centers.

My cousin Howard had by then established a busy neurosurgical/neurological practice in North Andover and gave me a half day a week that increased for a while to up to one and a half days a week, some of the time spent doing consults at the Northeast Rehab Hospital in Salem, New Hampshire. I'm sure he really didn't need me, but his practice generated

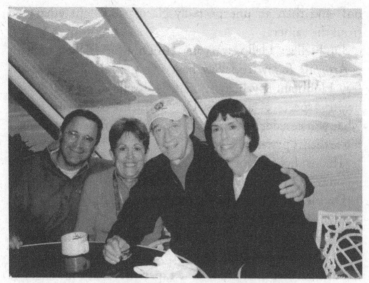

Fern, Jeff, Howard, and Naomi—Alaska Cruise

work for me too. I would be involved in New England Neurological, Howard's practice, including consulting at his rehab hospital, for the next fifteen years.

I did my best to market myself, giving talks to community groups and at hospitals. Matt Heller, a rheumatologist whose Lynnfield office was in the same building as mine, was an even more avid self-promoter than I was, and he asked me if I'd like to be a guest on his local cable TV show, *Arthritis Today*. I would be the "expert" on the psychological aspects of arthritic disease. I had never been on television before, but I figured "How hard can it be?"

On the day of the show, Matt took me to the studio and showed me the setup. After about a minute of prep he told me, "Don't forget. When the red light by the camera goes on, we're live."

We sat at a coffee table à la *Today Show*, the camera a few feet in front of us. The director signaled "Three, two, one . . .

on!" and then an unexpectedly glaring red light emanated from the camera.

Dr. Heller: "Hello, everyone. I'm Dr. Matt Heller, and this is *Arthritis Today*. Today we have a very special guest, Dr. Jeffrey Hoffman, psychiatrist, and we'll talk about the mental health aspects of arthritis. Dr. Hoffman, could you tell us what you consider the most important emotional issues facing arthritis patients?"

The red light seemed brighter, filling the room. Ten, twenty seconds go by. Nothing from Dr. Hoffman.

Dr. Heller: "Let me put it another way . . ."

That didn't work, either.

Afterward, Matt did his best to console me ("It happens to all of us. Don't worry about it."), but needless to say, there were no further invitations. The experience made me angry at myself. I felt that I should have been able to do the show and would have if I were better prepared. In fact, I had a number of more successful cable TV experiences, one of which was almost too successful.

I agreed to participate in a program sponsored by a local hospital and did a series of six half-hour TV interviews with its public relations person. In each one, I discussed the diagnosis and treatment of common problems in psychiatry: depression, anxiety, substance abuse, major mental illness, dementia, and attention-deficit disorder. They showed it over and over again, and a number of my patients commented that they had seen the shows and liked them, but I noticed that I had started getting fewer patients sent to me from a couple of my regular referral sources. I felt comfortable enough with one of them to ask if I had done anything wrong. "Oh no," he said, "but your TV series is like a minifellowship. I do my own psychiatry now."

Early practice years got busy fast, but I made my share of rookie mistakes.

Jeanie Farini was a very attractive woman in her midtwenties whom I first encountered when I was doing a consulting job at our local state hospital, Danvers State, where I was asked to give a second opinion. Jeanie was recovering from her most recent psychotic break. When I saw her, she was charming, flirtatious, and absolutely crazy. A few weeks later I got a call from her father, who asked me to take her on as a private patient. I agreed to do so, a decision that did neither of us any good.

Initially we established a good rapport, but inevitably she became very psychotic and required rehospitalization. My previous experiences had all been on established and well-organized inpatient units where I trained and in the air force. At this time, in my early practice, I wasn't on staff at a hospital with an inpatient unit where I would be able to personally care for Jeanie. The best I could do was J. B. Thomas Hospital in Peabody, Massachusetts. One of its medical units accepted nondangerous psychiatric patients, and it had a partial hospitalization program where the inpatients received day treatment during the week. I figured that I could fill in with seven-day-a-week therapy on my morning rounds.

Jeanie took her medications as far as the nurses could tell, but instead of improving, she seemed to be getting more psychotic. Specifically, she was developing a rip-roaring psychotic transference toward me, a process that a more experienced doctor would have anticipated and avoided by transferring her to a more traditional mental health unit. As the days went on, she projected her considerable paranoia directly to me, accusing me of "torturing her" and "mind-raping her twenty-four hours a day" and asking "how could I do this if I loved her?"

Eventually, Jeanie left the hospital against medical advice (ultimately a good move on her part) and wound up back at Danvers State. A few weeks later, I got a letter from Jeanie telling me that she forgave me for what I did to her in the hospital and that she was all better. She then went on to describe what she would like to do with me in intimate, romantic terms. Then in the second part of the letter, she described in bloody detail just how she'd like to dismember me, my most important member first. She signed the letter "All my love, Jeanie."

So, I sent a letter to Jeanie and her dad saying that as much as I liked Jeanie, it would be best if she found another doctor.

That was not quite the end of it. About three years later I was seeing a new patient, my last patient of the day, a prim, elderly, and depressed Lynnfield lady. From outside my office we heard a glass-piercing shriek, then the sound of the door opening, and there was Jeanie, running down my hallway, disheveled and screaming, "Dr. Hoffman! Please saaave me!" Following close behind was a Massachusetts state trooper and, huffing and puffing behind him was Jeanie's obese dad.

Jeanie had been in the back of a police vehicle with her father, in the process of being taken for an involuntary hospitalization, when the car was slowed by traffic on a highway half a mile away. She bolted from the car and ran to my office. I guess she forgave me after all.

Transference, roughly defined, refers to the feelings a patient has toward his or her doctor. The feelings might be anger, fear, desire to please, and, yes, sexual attraction. It can be an invaluable guide to what's going on in the patient and in the therapy and is always to be used in the patient's best interest. If you miss something, there can be consequences.

Cindy was a very attractive bipolar patient around thirty-five years old who was married to a much older man. She was often mildly hypomanic, even on lithium, but overall fairly stable. She often complained about her marriage and often said that she regretted not marrying someone closer to her age.

It was clear that Cindy was attracted to me, and she was a little flirtatious, but she was religious, a regular churchgoer, and, I thought, committed to her marriage and her treatment.

On one particular visit during the summer Cindy came in wearing a terrycloth beach robe, the kind with snaps in front. She said that she had just come from the beach and apologized for her attire. About ten minutes into the session Cindy stared at me for a second, then stood up and tore open the snaps on her robe, revealing a very skimpy and sexy Victoria Secret outfit, and exclaimed, "Dr. Hoffman, take me!"

Cindy looked great! This was not sexy, though. It was really scary.

I don't remember how I did it, but I managed to convince her to snap her robe shut and called her husband to come pick her up. He was surprisingly understanding, at least in front of me. She did later genuinely apologize, and I was able to continue to treat her after setting some explicit boundaries. Her marriage worked out.

Early practice was not all blunders and embarrassment; there were some real saves too.

Denise was another bipolar patient, albeit far less stable. She was lovely and well controlled when she was on her medication, but her condition could escalate in a frighteningly short time to a hypermanic state, a kind of agitated delirium that if untreated can be life-threatening.

Denise had missed a number of appointments, and I hadn't seen her in several months when I received a desperate phone call from her husband. He sounded like he was in tears. "Please, Dr. Hoffman, Denise is going to die. You've got to help her. She's at Danvers State Hospital; they won't treat her."

I asked, "What do you mean they won't treat her?"

"She's pregnant. They won't give her medication."

I told her husband that I was not on staff at Danvers and had no status there, but because she was committed there, he couldn't take her out. He begged me to come to the hospital even if only as a visitor.

The desperation in his voice told me that I had to do something, so I drove to the hospital, where he met me and took me to the exam room. There was Denise, tied to an examining table with four-point restraints, looking about ten months pregnant, red-faced, straining at her shackles, and screaming incoherently. It was apparent that if she wasn't sedated, she would blow out the baby like a cannonball as well as her placenta and most of her blood volume any second.

I asked to see the treating psychiatrist and politely introduced myself as her outpatient psychiatrist. I diplomatically suggested that Denise needed sedation pronto. The "doctor" answered, in thickly accented English, "No medication, lady pregnant."

I couldn't believe my ears and told him that if Denise weren't treated quickly, she and the baby would die and not in a pretty way. I suggested that if he didn't want to treat her, he could just leave the Haldol and Ativan out and leave the room. I'd be glad to give it to her myself.

Foreign doc. relented and treated Denise, and before too long she settled down, much to my relief and the relief and gratitude of her husband. She gave birth to a healthy boy about a week later.

My private practice years were divided into two parts of roughly equal length. In the first half of my career, I worked as a traditional psychiatrist and was very involved in many types of psychotherapy, including behavioral, marital, family, sexual dysfunction, and hypnosis, as well as traditional psychoanalytically oriented psychodynamic psychotherapy. At New England Neurological, I did biofeedback. And, of course, I practiced pharmacotherapy, which became my focus during the latter part of my career. In general I hospitalized my own inpatients, trying to avoid any further Jeanie Farini experiences.

One of the most challenging character types to treat is someone with borderline personality disorder. Such people are highly impulsive with poorly regulated emotions, and they experience chaotic interpersonal relationships because of persistent fears of abandonment as well as extreme swings between idealization and devaluation of others. In the 1970s and 1980s the treatment of choice was long-term psychotherapy, a minimum of two to three times per week for several years. The idea was to re-create the patient's emotional distortions in therapy, allowing those feelings to develop toward the therapist (transference) in a safe environment where they could be gradually examined and corrected.

Nancy was a woman of about thirty-two when I first started to treat her. She lived with her mother, with whom she had a tempestuous relationship. Nancy had undergone multiple hospitalizations after overdoses or incidents of cutting her arms following arguments with her mother or after brief failed relationships. Nancy presented to me dressed in a shabby fashion, in drab colors. She cut her hair short and unstylishly, wore no makeup, and had moderate acne. She hardly ever smiled and always seemed angry. Altogether, she had the look of a chronic patient in a state hospital. She almost seemed to be trying to make herself unattractive. She presented with a litany of complaints about her mother and told me that she herself was always being disappointed by others.

I mostly listened, and inevitably she began to grow comfortable with me. Why couldn't others in her life be as understanding as me, she'd ask. With borderlines, though, you don't have to wait too long for the other shoe to drop, and she would test me with frequent middle-of-the-night crisis calls and demands on my time that I could not possibly fulfill. Sure enough, her idealization of me turned to disappointment and rage followed by overdoses, which were my "fault."

The greatest challenge with borderlines is managing your own countertransference—that is, negative feelings toward patients—and not acting on them inappropriately (e.g., refusing to take telephone calls). The therapist's capacity to contain his or her feelings toward the patient despite multiple provocations in a safe environment was considered to be and was a healing experience.

While trying to set some limits with Nancy, I continued to see her regularly. Sometimes the sessions consisted of me listening to her opinion of how lousy a therapist I was and how I was wasting her time. But she almost never missed an appointment.

About three years into treatment, she made reference to the fact that she was picked up at a bar by a guy named Walter. I was concerned that this would turn into another brief, destructive relationship and would end in a suicide attempt. For some reason, she continued to see Walter but often talked about him in demeaning ways.

"He's such a wuss. Why does he put up with me? Why doesn't he stand up to me? How can he stand me?" She never seemed to have much good to say about Walter, but somehow she stuck with him (as she stuck with me).

So gradually that I barely noticed it, Nancy began to look better. She was wearing a touch of makeup, and her clothes and haircut—were they actually getting a little more stylish? When she talked about Walter she was still somewhat critical, but now she seemed to be able to laugh about it. And the overdoses stopped.

Because over time I was able to tolerate and accept Nancy, she became better able to accept herself. Apparently it went similarly with Walter, and she became able to tolerate someone's love without unrealistic expectations, which would invariably sabotage things. They married eventually. I hope things went well for them—I bet they did.

This type of therapy was challenging for me; it took a very long time and tested my abilities to their limit. Today, borderlines are more often treated by a method called dialectical behavioral therapy, which is much briefer and often quite effective. It does *not* focus on transference or countertransference at all and instead helps patients deal with real-life distortions in real time and also helps them evaluate the consequences of their self-destructive impulsivity. Most important, it helps them better handle and contain the emotions that lead to their difficulties. All current effective modern psychotherapies are more targeted than in the past and are most effectively combined with medications. Psychotherapy has not left mental health care—it has just gotten more efficient and effective.

This is not to say that psychoanalytic thinking has not contributed many useful concepts to the understanding of the human mind and the processes that occur in a psychotherapeutic or any doctor patient relationship: transference, countertransference, resistance (the mind's unconscious reluctance to change), and the unconscious itself (events occurring in the mind out of a person's awareness but affecting his or her thoughts and behavior), and many others.

The notion of therapeutic boundaries, a psychoanalytic concept about treatment, is one of great importance in any patient-treater relationship not just for psychiatrists but also for all doctors and caregivers. It helps define the parameters beyond which any therapeutic relationship ought not to go if it is to be successful and ethical.

Most obvious are strictures against any type of sexual interaction or inappropriate touching between patient and doctor. Social friendship or any type of business relationship is also out of bounds. The doing of favors and the giving or receiving of gifts apart from a holiday greeting card is also verboten, but . . .

Danielle was a thirty-something single woman who came to me for the treatment of anxiety and depression and for psychotherapy with problems in her personal relationships, including the tendency to allow people to take advantage of her.

I treated Danielle with an antidepressant and a low dose benzodiazepine (a medication in the Valium family) on which she responded well. She was able to taper off the antidepressant but continued on the low-dose benzo, which she seemed to use appropriately to good effect.

However, Danielle gradually began to admit that she was dependent on alcohol, using it regularly and sometimes excessively. At this point many psychiatrists would attempt to taper the benzodiazepine, which does not generally work well with alcohol abusers. I tried to do so unsuccessfully.

Danielle had several jobs in order to make ends meet, and one of them was for the Red Sox at the ticket office of Fenway Park. Once she asked me, "Doc. do you ever go to Red Sox games?" I was and still am a Red Sox fan and took the bait. "Yes, once in a while with my kids." Danielle then commented, "Next time you come, stop by my ticket window. We always hold back a few great seats for VIPs who show up at the last minute. If they're available, we can do an exchange."

The next time I was at Fenway with Dan or Jess, I came to Danielle's window to exchange my lousy right field seats for seats behind home plate. I made several subsequent visits with Dan or Jess or both, trading for home plate, dugout, or a special protected VIP section on the second deck. I always paid for the cost difference, but of course the "gift" was access to fabulous seats that I could never have gotten on my own.

Was this an inappropriate gift? Absolutely! Was I allowing myself to take advantage of Danielle, one of the very issues for which she came to me for help? For certain! I also continued her on the low-dose benzos, rationalizing that she never overused them and that in a small percentage of cases it may be appropriate to continue them (if this is ever so, it is only if a patient has had extended sobriety and only in limited quantities). To what extent did the better baseball tickets adversely affect my treatment of her?

I regret this and hope that it ultimately did not do Danielle great harm. But we really enjoyed those fabulous seats.

However, for me, while interesting to do, psychotherapy was time-consuming, and insurance paid poorly for it. Also, by the early 1990s psychopharmacology was a burgeoning field and interesting in its own right. With some regret, I decided to phase out my psychotherapy practice. I had a family to raise and educate. So, I began accepting new patients for pharmacotherapy only.

As a part-time doctor at Howard's New England Neurological practice, I was privy to his numerous medical project investment opportunities: CT scan, MRI, PET scan, industrial medicine, nursing homes. A few failed, but most were successful. If there was a moneymaking opportunity, Howard sniffed it out. He was as much medical entrepreneur as neurosurgeon.

The format for each new opportunity was always the same. Howard would gather his medical minions, describe the new project in detail and all the ways it could fail, and tell us that we could easily lose all our money. He'd say how much he needed to raise and invite us all to "Call out a number." This would be followed by the group falling all over itself to throw money at Howard like it was confetti.

Howard's most spectacularly successful project was the Northeast Rehab Hospital, which was followed by other highly successful rehab hospitals as well as over twenty physical therapy practices, all with the same partnership. My own modest involvement, based on what Fern and I thought we could afford, turned out to be the gift that keeps on giving and has been a nice income enhancer.

When we were both thirty-two, Fern and I finally felt that we were secure enough to shop for a house. We set an arbitrary maximum, which turned out to be less than we could afford, and after looking and dithering, we settled on a pretty but impractical house on a steep hill in the St. John's Prep area of Danvers, a beautiful new neighborhood. The house was located atop a steep horseshoe driveway. It looked great in the summer when we bought it, but for half the year it was an icy and dangerous cliff.

We were lucky to have good neighbors, and the best of them lived next door, PJ and Laurie Curran. PJ was from Ireland and had a fantastic brogue that I'm sure he cultivates as a tour guide in Boston and Salem, charming international visitors. Laurie also has a unique musical voice and a caring personality to go with. Except for one tiny dispute, we got along famously for years. One morning I awoke to hear the buzz of an electric saw and went outside, where PJ was busily cutting down one of my favorite trees, which was on the border of our properties. I was a tree person, PJ was "a let the sunlight in" person. and we disagreed as to whose property the tree belonged. We agreed to jointly pay for a surveyor, who confirmed that it was my tree. PJ apologized and cut the tree into firewood for us, the only dispute in more than thirty years settled.

The Currans had two children: Sarah, who was about Jessica's age, and Brendan, a few years younger. As parents PJ and Laurie were considerably stricter than we were, particularly in monitoring their kids' TV watching: no R-rated cable TV allowed. On that matter Fern and I set essentially no limits, so Sarah became a secret TV-watching buddy of Jessica's, binging on verboten HBO. I think that we and the Currans pretended not to notice.

Brendan was a little grown-up in a child's costume from the time he could talk. He was unusually articulate before the age of three, addressing us respectfully as "Dr. and Mrs. Hoffman," but was never shy about expressing himself or his needs. He seemed hilariously unintimidated by adults. It came as no surprise that he grew up to become an outspoken advocate of many human rights causes and uses his voice as a pastor in a nearby church.

soccer and tennis
ead, a Jewish day
ur ski weekends
o go to Hebrew

y Ralph Waldo
the untamed
ous privacy of
replace watch-
ter storms as
io announce-
chial schools

school who
end of ski-
d to enjoy.

e was a group of
ouples Club, and

iching and became
losed my practice.
mine, and she did
running my practice
rance companies and
ionate and caring with
iestly) while raising our
me care and devotion.
ind extremely competent.
her. She is a detail person,
e. I'm better at major deci-
mentation. We complement
e tennis court). I'm lucky to

on January 24, 1978, between
ortunately, Fern's parents were
ents through the infamous Mas-
Dan's fetal heart rate kept falling
or, and it was touch and go on the
ie end, he came out the usual way
locked firmly around his umbilical
mittent low heart rate. Did he think
n airplane?

brain damage, Dan turned out to be
was reasonably easy as babies go. He
id young and became a know-it-all even
fted student from the start and a better
himself credit for.

years and three months later on April 24,
ssier as an infant, smart but shy, and defi-
tive. She was the athlete of the family and

became a graceful skier and an outstanding
player.

We sent the kids to a school in Marbleh
school called Hillel Academy, largely so that
would not be disrupted by our kids having
school on the weekends.

When I was a schoolboy we read a poem b
Emerson called "The Snowstorm," evoking
beauty of a winter storm. The phrase "a tumult
storm" conveyed the image of sitting by a cozy fi
ing the wild beauty from a safe place. I loved wi
a child, especially if followed by the morning rad
ment "All Philadelphia public, private, and paro
are closed."

Later, I envied the rich kids at college and med
made the twelve-hour trek to Vermont for a wee
ing and all kinds of fun that the well-to-do seeme

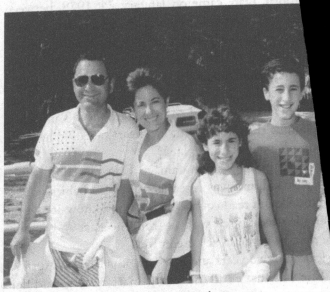

Young Family

So, in our late twenties and living in an apartment outside Philly when Fern noticed an ad in a local newspaper for a "Learn to Ski" course given at a local junior college, we both saw it as a great opportunity.

The course was given at Chad's Peak, a tiny ski hill with wretched conditions. The hill on which we learned was more often icy than snowy. We were taught by the so-called graduated length method, starting on very short skis and graduating to the long boards that were used at that time.

I wasn't much of a natural, falling frequently and full of bruises but grimly determined. The only instruction I recall was "Jeff, relax, its supposed to be fun." But Fern and I became intermediate skiers, and the following year we took our first ski trip to Heavenly Valley at Lake Tahoe. It was heavenly, skiing beautiful winter scenes to exhaustion and being a part of it. Skiing remained a part of our lives for the next forty years.

We loved ski weekends. We went to a number of different New England ski areas, but eventually we decided to buy our own place at the Sunday River Ski Resort near Bethel, Maine, a one-bedroom condo with its own wood-burning fireplace. We owned the place for twenty years and spent as many winter weekends and vacation weeks there as possible. Dan and Jessica were enrolled in the freestyle ski program, which they both liked, and Fern and I were involved in adult social ski groups. Our kids became experts, and we got good enough to enjoy ourselves without breaking anything.

Our good friends from Danvers, Ben Polan, a dentist, and Bonnie Polan, a teacher, also bought a place at Sunday River. Their daughter, Briana, is close in age to Jess, and the two girls had a bit of a rivalry in the ski program. In one competition Briana came in seventh and Jessica eighth, undistinguished enough, but when Bonnie decided to put a little blurb about these great accomplishments in Hillel's (the kid's school)

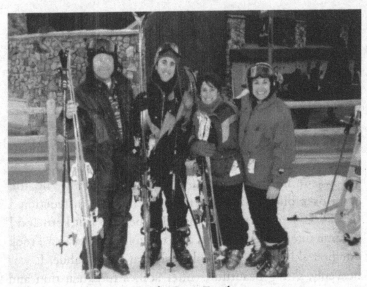

Sunday River Family

monthly newsletter, Fern almost had a stroke and fractured their friendship. Fern got over it—eventually. We loved the Polans, but we could be a little competitive with them.

We skied with another family, the Keenholtzes, Steve and Roberta, a local internist and a recovery nurse whose oldest daughter, Erica, an assertive little pistol, was a classmate and friend of Jessica's. When Erica stayed with us at Sunday River, they would either giggle or fight all night, at times requiring us to separate them at three or four in the morning so we could ski the next day, when, invariably, we'd be exhausted and they'd be buddies again.

Jessica was shy and socially fearful. She eventually transferred to public school, where she stayed through the tenth grade. In her early years we had to cajole her to study, but at some point early in high school she did an about-face and became a compulsive studier and was extremely neurotic about grades. To this day I'm not entirely sure what that was about.

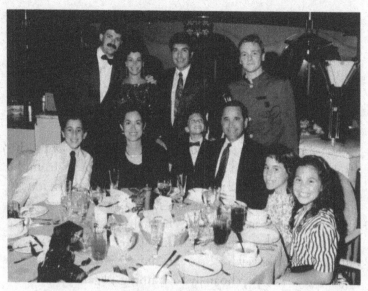

Hoffman and Polans Cruise

Jessica's athleticism was one of her strong suits. Aside from being a graceful skier, she was also a soccer talent and earned her a position as a midfielder on the town's traveling soccer team for her age group. I was involved a little as an assistant coach for the team, and I loved it. One year the team made the state finals, as much or more of a thrill for us parents as for the kids. Jessica was still shy, but her teammates accepted and respected her.

People have often asked me whether my psychiatric training helped me as a parent (what they may have been thinking is that his kids are at least as messed up as ours). Frankly, neither my flaws nor good attributes as a parent had much to do in any direct way with my psychiatric background. Psychiatric residencies don't typically include parenting training (maybe they should).

It is true that in marital therapy, parenting issues come up all the time in the context of serious marital problems or coping with parental stress while suffering from depression, severe anxiety, schizophrenia, or the many other mental health problems that we treat.

Between myself and Fern, I tended to be the more permissive and she the structured parent. But when the kids got me really angry I could yell, swear, and occasionally swat bottoms with the best of them.

The stereotype of the aloof, totally in control cool psychiatric parent has lasted surprisingly long and comes from the distorted view that the restraint required to be shown in psychoanalytic therapy is often transferred to the home front. Even fifty years ago when psychoanalysis held much more sway, I doubt that most psychiatric parents acted that way, but woe to the kids whose parents did.

(To be clear, psychoanalytic training began toward the end of psychiatric residencies or immediately after and was originally only open to psychiatrically trained MDs. Until the 1960s most ambitious psychiatrists went on for this training, which consisted of many courses on Freudian theory and technique, psychoanalyzing your own patients at a clinic under the supervision of a senior psychoanalyst, and, most important, your own psychoanalysis by a training analyst, a lengthy and expensive process that took many years.)

Pure psychoanalysis occurred four to six hours per week, with the patient literally lying on a couch not seeing the analyst, who sat behind. The so-called pure gold of psychoanalysis requires that the patient not see the analyst and the analyst not in the least betray his or her emotional feelings toward the patient. This was not because the analyst had none but because doing so would prevent the formation of a transference neurosis. The theory stated that over time the patient would transfer his or her neurosis onto the person of the analyst, where the feelings and conflicts toward the doctor could be gradually and safely dealt with (analyzed). Eventually the conflicts would be resolved, mental health would be improved, and the patient would be freed from the impeding neurosis that originally brought him or her into treatment.

This required restraint particularly from unnecessary inter-action with the patient and is called therapeutic abstinence; analysts train for years to be skilled at this. It is an interesting theory. Its only problem is that the opposite is true. Many years ago a psychiatrist named Jerome Frank wrote an impor-tant book about psychotherapy titled *Persuasion and Healing*.

It included a number of scientific studies showing that the most effective psychotherapies occurred when patients felt that their therapists were actively engaged, faced their patients and actually cared what happened to them, and were not aloof seeming and distant regardless of the theoretical rationale. Later studies have confirmed Frank's views.

So, whatever one may have thought of me as a parent, no one would accuse me of being aloof. On many winter Friday nights after a hard week for all of us, we would pile into our SUV to make the three-hour trip to Sunday River, all of us tired and often irritable. The kids would invariably quar-rel, yelling at each other in the backseat. Family lore had it that when Grandpa Harry drove and the Feinberg kids were screaming in the backseat, with his 6′ frame and long arms he could smack all three in one stroke. When I tried to do it on the way to skiing with my 5′7″ height and short arms, they barely made it over the back of the front seat, to the vast amusement of my kids, who would say, "You're not trying to be Grandpa Harry are you? Grow some arms."

Once when Jess was in her teens and got me really angry about something, I threw a remote control at her, which for-tunately missed. I felt terrible and apologized profusely, but Jess would have none of it. She ran to the phone and said, "I'm going to call the child abuse hotline," which existed in Massachusetts. As she picked up the phone, I pointed out to her that they were really efficient and that a social worker would come by the house probably immediately (I had no idea whatsoever) and place her in foster care, and I told her, "Remember, no skiing, no Sunday River, no private school, no more soccer team," at which point Jess put down the receiver.

In social situations, folks are sometimes intimidated when in small talk they learn that I'm a psychiatrist and make comments such as "Doctor, you're not going to analyze me are you?"

I usually politely joke back that "the taxi meter is off for the night" or "not without your insurance card," but what I'm usually thinking is "What makes you think you're so important that I'd want to waste a perfectly good martini and social evening analyzing you?"

Living in New England near my cousins Naomi, Howard, Howard's daughters, David (who settled in Gloucestert to practice law with Irving), and Uncle Irving and his wife Lia, we never needed an excuse to throw a party. Between bar and bat mitzvahs, graduations, and weddings we were always celebrating something at someone's house. Fern and Naomi alternated having Thanksgivings, which were traditional New England celebrations with a generous table of turkey and fixings. My parents were there and occasionally Fern's as well as dates and later spouses and grandkids. When our kids were growing up things tended to be a little dressier, which added to the holiday feeling. Irving and Lia and David and his wife Janice came. Irving had met Lia on one of his trips to Europe. She was a German lady several years younger than he, and he married for the first time when he was fifty-nine years old. They both passed away shortly after their twenty-fifth anniversary. Irving's sisters, mother, and Aunt Miriam thought that it would be practical for them to buy a condo, but neither would have any of that. Lia fancied herself a continental sophisticate, and they bought a beautiful large old wooden totally impractical New England home, with a large porch and lots of land. In Irving's sixties and seventies they had killer parties at their house, which Fern and I enjoyed immensely. And for a time they felt that they were in the midst of the Gloucester social scene, as Lia was a charming hostess, with her love of fun and her German accent. As they aged, the needs of the house kind of overwhelmed them.

Summers we had annual Fourth of July family outings at Howard's house on the ocean, David's house in Gloucester, or our house in Danvers. The highlight was usually a full-scale New England clam bake with steamers, as much lobster as you could eat, and all the usual accoutrements. Summer being nicer weather, they were often attended by friends or family from Philly, Cleveland, Hawaii, and Germany.

While our families didn't socialize beyond these gatherings, what was noteworthy was that people actually seemed to get along and enjoy each other's company.

In 1990 it was time to begin planning for Dan's bar mitzvah, a year of nonstop partying for all Jewish boys and girls of that age. We were in the process of remodeling our house in Danvers, an exhausting project requiring us to move the whole family out for three months. We moved into the same small apartment Fern and I had lived in fourteen years before. Living in a relatively small space while a less than fully reliable contractor did the remodeling job was stressful, but the finished product was better and roomier; there was a two-car garage and a safer driveway as well as enormous changes to the house, and it was finished in time for the bar mitzvah.

Learning the bar mitzvah material was easy for Dan, but actually standing in front of all his friends and relatives was another matter. From the time he woke up on the morning of the service until literally seconds before it was his moment to chant, he kept pitifully repeating, with a look of anguished pleading, "Don't make me do it. Don't make me do it." I thought about my own experience, how I'd frozen in the TV studio when the red light was turned on, and how I'd help

Dan if he got up there in front of everybody and nothing came out. Once we pushed him onto the bimah, though, his performance was flawless. Expecting him to give a speech on top of that, however, was too much to ask, so that was my job.

A year before we had attended the bar mitzvah of Dan's classmate Danny Gelb, whose dad, an attorney, gave a speech for his son. I thought at the time that I'd like to do that and wrote a speech, which I memorized and delivered after the service right before the lunch, and it came off pretty well.

After that I became a sort of the poet laureate of our family and through the years made a hobby of writing poems for family and friends on various occasions, some of which might have been entertaining.

That weekend we hosted our friends and relatives as well as many of our parents' friends, who had come up from Philadelphia. We had a Sunday brunch at our house, the only part of the weekend when Fern and I could really relax.

Jessica's bat mitzvah almost wasn't. She had zero interest in having one at all, let alone a traditional event like Dan's. However, a friend had taken his family on a bar mitzvah tour to Israel, which was how we learned that there were companies that arranged family tours, including a ceremony at the Western Wall or at Masada—the site of a famous battle in which a bunch of Jewish religious fanatics committed mass suicide, women and children included, making them all martyrs for the faith. This sounded perfect for Jessica. She couldn't care less, but all a kid had to do was a line or two of Torah to officially be a part of our tribe. While not enthusiastic, Jessica went along with it.

It turned out to be a fabulous trip. I had never been to Israel, and I fell in love with the pure vitality of this uniquely Jewish land. For two weeks we traveled with several families of similar makeup, visiting numerous archaeological and biblical sites as well as the sights of modern Israel. We toured the West Bank, the Golan Heights, Tel Aviv, Haifa, and, of course, Jerusalem and the Western Wall. The early-morning ceremony at Masada was simple but moving, and you felt a sense of the continuity of the Jewish people. The visit to Yad Vashem, the Holocaust memorial, was sad but compelling.

As a result of this trip, Fern and I became committed to the importance of the survival of Israel and have become avid supporters of the American Israel Public Affairs Committee, the organization that promotes the ongoing special relationship between the United States and Israel. The need for Israel as a permanent refuge for the Jewish people is pretty obvious to me. Anti-Semitism is alive and well in the world. Anyone who doesn't think that there are millions of people alive today who would enthusiastically volunteer to complete Hitler's work just hasn't been paying attention.

Also, Israel and the Jewish people have flooded the world with gifts of scientific discovery, jurisprudence, and the arts wildly disproportionate to their numbers. I've often wondered why that is and have a little theory (completely unproven) of my own. I think that it has to do with millennia of Talmud study. The Talmud is a collection of laws and commentary written by rabbis over the centuries, a body of work that is the basis for governing all aspects of traditional Jewish life and practice. It is extensive and complex, and studying it successfully requires intellectual brilliance and creativity.

Jews have traditionally honored and revered their most able Talmud scholars above everyone else, and the best Talmud students frequently had marriages arranged with the daughters of the most brilliant rabbis. This just might have created an evolutionary bottleneck favoring the birth of a relatively large proportion of highly capable Talmud scholars instead of hugely muscled men. Traditional Jewish culture has favored this unusual form of selection for thousands of years. I don't know what it is about the capacity to do well at Talmud study that could have resulted in later generations excelling in science, let alone the arts, but I suspect that it is there. The relationship of Talmud study to the capacity to be a great lawyer and judge is more obvious. Later generations might or might not continue Talmud study, but they pass on their abilities to their offspring and the world.

Also, if as Thomas Edison is supposed to have said genius is 2 percent inspiration and 98 percent perspiration—by which he meant patience, persistence, and attention to detail—then what other tradition inculcates this better than one that in its traditional form insists on meticulous daily adherence to the hundreds (613 to be exact) of laws governing all aspects of Jewish life?

Interestingly, the Jewish communities most likely to survive in the future are the most observant ones, and the most prolific of these are the ultraorthodox. They're the ones who will breed new generations of Talmud talent. Frankly, this is most likely to continue in Israel if the country continues to maintain its theocratic basis, with policies that foster support of the ultraorthodox.

We've been fortunate enough to enjoy other great travels over the years, mostly with university groups. We've been all over Europe, and we've been to China and the Great Wall, where Dan was taking a year off from college to work in marketing and practice speaking Mandarin, the easy language he took at Columbia. We've been to Machu Pichu in Peru. We went to Rio to meet Jessica's new boyfriend, Bruno, a Jewish med student and her future husband, an all-around great, goofy guy, and to South Africa, where we got to take pictures up close (very close) of lions, rhinos, giraffes, gazelles, and all of those *National Geographic* African beasts at Kreuger National Park. In Ireland we learned traditional Irish drinking songs, with which we still entertain ourselves, and we've been all over Italy, because Italy is great, as well as Greece, England, and many others lands.

In her sophomore year at Danvers High School, Jess was all-conference in tennis and doing okay academically, but she began to campaign intensely for us to send her to Gould Academy, a boarding school in Bethel, Maine, near Sunday River. Many of the Gould kids were involved in her freestyle skiing program, and she had come to be friends with a number of them. I was totally against sending my daughter away to boarding school and put my foot down. Besides, wasn't Gould a school for hyperactive misfits and future ski bums? Jess enrolled for her junior year and went on to graduate from Gould.

I admit that it turned out to be a good choice for Jess, and the school was much more impressive academically than I had expected. She made a number of close friends there and got into trouble a few times (unauthorized use of our condo), and she was all-conference in tennis and soccer and also established herself as a library nerd. She graduated in the top ten and got into the highly competitive physical therapy program at Northeastern University.

Dan was another story. He was pretty much an outstanding student from the start and won lots of awards at Hillel. St. John's Prep, our local academic Catholic boys' school, was just around the corner from us. We sent him there because it was convenient and academically more than enough challenge for "smarty pants." About 10 percent of the students were Jewish, and Dan did not mind going even though he was a bit of a wreck freshman year. He graduated salutatorian, and watching him give his graduation speech was one of the most sublimely proud moments of my life. He was also a National Merit scholar. He could have gone to any university in the country, and we visited the best in the East, but Columbia and New York City called to him, and that is where he went.

In the late 1980s I was becoming restless, discontent with my practice in Massachusetts. We considered moving to another part of the country, and an opportunity came up in

Gastonia, North Carolina, a town sixty miles west of Charlotte where the cost of living was much less than in the Northeast and the weather was better. A hospital was looking for a medical director of a seventy-bed psychiatric unit, embedded in a four hundred–bed general hospital. Fern and I flew down for two days of meetings and interviews at the hospital, and I also met with the principal of the local private school and families from the local temple. I was offered the job, which included the opportunity to set up my own practice.

At the same time one of our local hospitals, Salem Hospital, was expanding its own mental health unit, and joining there would give me the opportunity to admit my patients to a well-established psychiatric unit.

Whichever position I chose, my days at New England Neurological were ending. I was grateful to Howard, but traveling to New Hampshire and Andover, Massachusetts, while maintaining a practice on the North Shore was just too scattered.

Ultimately I decided to stay in Massachusetts and joined the staff of Salem Hospital.

On the way home from a vacation in Bermuda, our plane was caught in an electrical storm over JFK Airport in New York. The plane was ultimately rerouted to Washington, DC, but first we were stacked up for what seemed like hours, and while we were circling the plane was hit by lightning. The plane shook and the lights went out, followed by the loudest thunderclap I'd ever heard.

Two days later my ears began to ring, a constant high-pitched and fairly loud sound that wouldn't go away. Evaluations by a neurologist and an ear, nose, and throat doctor didn't help much. I was told that I had high-pitch hearing loss and a noise injury. No one could tell me when or if the tinnitus would ever subside. I became anxious, depressed, and irritable, and I had difficulty concentrating on my work. Fern and I finally flew out to the Health Sciences Center at the University of Oregon in

Portland, where they had an internationally famous center for the evaluation and treatment of tinnitus.

They couldn't cure me, but they prescribed maskers, devices that are worn like hearing aids. They emit a soft, pleasant, high-pitched "Shhh" sound that is supposed to mask the ringing during the day. They worked somewhat well. For nighttime, they created audiotapes of white noise the same frequency as my tinnitus, which worked very well, and I could finally get some decent sleep.

But the anxiety and depression persisted.

There were many good psychiatrists in the North Shore, but Howard Levy was the best. He was a true doctor's doctor as well as a personal friend. I asked to meet with him for a visit or two for a brief consultation. Brief stretched to weeks, then months and years. The tinnitus never left, but I haven't cared about it for years. Howard was a great psychiatrist, friend, and listener who with great skill and compassion helped me get through my struggles with tinnitus and its concomitant anxiety and depression. Many other issues arose, and he became this psychiatrist's psychiatrist. We had been friends before, but our social relationship ended. But he was always a friend to me, just in a different way.

Those years were extremely busy for me professionally. I was never much of a joiner or an organization person, and aside from the committee memberships required for staff privileges, my professional life was about maintaining my own practice. But Salem Hospital was looking to contract with the psychiatric staff as a group to take over psychiatric care on the mental health unit, the addictive disease unit, the partial hospitalization program, and psychiatric consultation at North Shore Children's Hospital and the psych ER, providing services for patients all over northeastern Massachusetts.

This interested me, and for a number of years I was president of the corporation (Psychiatric Physicians, PC) contracted to provide these services, a group that consisted of twenty local psychiatrists. My hope was to eventually convince this herd of cats to come together in one practice, a move that would have made economic and political sense. We brought in a practice consultant to advise us on its feasibility and how we would go about it. Unfortunately, the guys were too entrenched in their own practices and ways of doing things, and it never got off the ground.

However, I did manage to negotiate the terms of our relationship. We got good fee-for-service rates for all individual services without having to bill, which was Salem's responsibility. We had bimonthly business meetings, which generated lots of uncompensated and underappreciated work for me.

Eventually when the contract lapsed, we went our separate ways. But of the entire group, the person with whom I was most compatible, both personally and in style of practice style, was Bruce Goldberg (who had been the vice president of Psychiatric Physicians, PC). We moved to a new office in Danvers together, sharing office space and equipment.

I stopped hospital practice altogether in 1998. For the rest of my years in Massachusetts, I worked as an office-based psychopharmacologist. Bruce and I hired therapists from time to time or referred psychotherapy out.

Malpractice

Nobody wants to be sued. We try to be careful and meet the best standards of care. Psychiatrists are sued infrequently, but it happens. It happened to me once, and I hope it never happens again.

Jennie was a woman in her thirties with bipolar disorder whom I treated for a number of years. She seemed to require somewhat higher doses of lithium than usual to maintain mood stabilization, and I did routine blood monitoring of her lithium level and other studies, which showed levels a little higher than usual but nowhere near toxic. She had marital problems and was a smoker and marijuana user. She missed one of her visits late in the year, and I did not hear from her for a few months after that.

Then one afternoon, she came to my office in the middle of a busy day demanding a copy of her medical records. I told her I didn't have time to copy them right then and there, but if she sent me a request, I would send them to whoever she wanted.

Over the next few months, I got a series of requests from two Boston law offices and two local attorneys demanding the records. One was in the form of a subpoena informing me that I was being sued for malpractice.

Apparently, several weeks before Jennie had been hospitalized for pneumonia, went into septic shock, and was comatose for a number of days. During that time, she developed acute renal failure. She fully recovered but blamed all of it on my "mismanagement" of her lithium. My initial reaction was a combination of fear and anger. As far as I was concerned, the suit was frivolous.

The Massachusetts Medical Society apparently disagreed, and its board allowed the suit to proceed.

Peter Knight, my insurance lawyer, was recommended to me by (who else?) my cousin Howard, who had used him from time to time to defend suits against neurologists or neurosurgeons in his group. He considered Peter the best.

Peter was a tall (at least 6'5") patrician-looking man who felt that my former patient had absolutely no case. He told me that the Massachusetts Medical Society had a very low threshold for letting cases proceed and that I should try not to worry about it—easy for him to say. He also pointed out that these cases often drag on for years and that I should just live my life and continue my practice.

I studied the details of Jennie's hospitalization thoroughly and reviewed her years of treatment as completely as I was able. I participated in a number of preparatory meetings with Peter, culminating with my deposition by her lawyer, her fifth. I had experts, she had experts, and it was amazing how different experts could interpret facts so differently.

My case was scheduled to go to trial in September 2011, and I was told to set aside a week for the ordeal. Two weeks prior to going to trial, I got a call from Peter. Jennie had offered to settle for fifty thousand dollars. I realized how costly and difficult a trial could be and told Peter that I really didn't want to be a defendant but that there was no way I'd agree to settle. Jennie's illness wasn't my fault. I was ready to go.

Peter—somewhat to my surprise, because I thought lawyers liked to settle—said, "I'm glad you feel that way. I was obligated to present you with the offer, but I'd have been really pissed if you had taken it."

Two days later Peter called back. "Good news, Jeff. She dropped the case, with prejudice," he told me, which meant that she could not refile it.

On reflection, I figured that after running through a number of lawyers who saw no merit in her case, she found one who made a living filing lots of malpractice suits, hoping there would always be a few who'd settle to avoid going to court.

Fern and I spent trial week in Nantucket. It beat the hell out of being a defendant.

Suicide

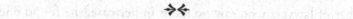

IN A PSYCHIATRIST'S professional life, there is no worse event than the suicide of a patient. Other doctors may lose patients to illnesses they treat, but if you're a psychiatrist, even if it really isn't your fault, it always feels like it is. For the families, it's always a painful loss that seems like it shouldn't have been.

Mabel was in her midfifties, a vital and usually cheerful woman. She was happily married and had a lovely family, with four adult children and several grandchildren.

For absolutely no apparent reason, this picture was marred when she had developed severe and unexplained panic attacks a few years earlier. These were sudden overwhelming episodes of anxiety that came and went randomly. They were the worst I'd ever seen in any patient. Medical evaluation failed to show any organic cause for her episodes, and psychotherapy, relaxation training, selective serotonin reuptake inhibitors, tricyclic antidepressants, all helpful in some patients, were useless for Mabel.

Antianxiety agents weren't useful either except for Xanax, which at high dosages took the edge off Mabel's panic attacks but still did not prevent them.

In desperation, we agreed to a trial on monoamine oxidase (MAO) inhibitors, which were reported to help with severe panic attacks but were much less frequently used because of their many dietary and medication-interaction restrictions. If you mix an MAO inhibitor with the wrong food or medication, you risk a hypertensive crisis. Even if precautions are followed, low blood pressure with severe lightheadedness is a common side effect.

For Mabel, the MAO inhibitor, Nardil specifically, was a miracle drug. The panic attacks went away completely, but she was left with constant lightheadedness and dizziness, and she hated taking it. She would often skip doses, whereupon the panic attacks returned. She would self-treat with Xanax, which only gave her fair relief.

Late one evening, Mabel called. The panic attacks were back and were worse than ever. She had stopped the Nardil a few days before. "They're awful," she told me, crying on the phone. "I feel like I want to kill myself."

I had no appointment for the next day but set one up for the morning after. I put her back on high doses of Xanax temporarily and told her to call me the next day if the attacks didn't improve. As she had never been previously suicidal, I hoped to get her through the crisis. What I didn't know is that she owned a shotgun.

The next morning I got a call from our local ER. Mabel had blown her brains out.

I couldn't believe that this once happy, vital woman, who had so many good things in her life, had chosen to end it. I questioned myself for not having hospitalized Mabel immediately and blamed myself for my judgment. What seemed like a reasonable delay ended in disaster.

I contacted the family, and they agreed to meet me in the ER. It was the longest drive of my life. The family was in so much pain and was so angry. I let them vent, and I think they realized that I was genuinely in pain too. But then they asked me to leave the meeting room so they could be alone, which I gladly did. I never saw them again.

Dan at College

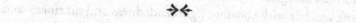

COLUMBIA UNIVERSITY, the "urban, intellectual Ivy" (at least according to Columbia's marketing material) stuffed into Manhattan's noisy, crowded, and always lively Upper West Side, was where Dan spent his college and med school years. I couldn't figure out why a kid who could have gone to Harvard, a school of similar demographics but superior cachet, would choose Columbia. But Dan loved the idea of being in New York City and, truthfully, putting a little distance between himself and home. His freshman dorm had all the amenities of an urban slum, but Dan seemed happy from the start, living there with a bunch of smart, fast-talking undergraduates with at least the veneer of self-confidence. Everyone seemed to speak the same "don't try to get a word in edgewise" rapid-fire patois.

We visited fairly often, and eventually I got to the point of liking the city as long as the visits lasted no more than a few days, after which the dirt, noise, and inflated cost of everything set me longing to return to peaceful, boring Danvers. But we enjoyed meeting Dan's college friends and attending activities at Columbia. We saw our share of shows and museums, but visiting with our son was for me always the best part of being in New York.

Dan started as a biochem major. I saw in him a future MD/PhD type, and I had visions of him becoming a Nobel-winning scientist. A summer research job after his freshman year convinced him that he was not a lab guy, though, and he switched his major to economics and math, a move I thought impulsive.

So, I switched my fantasy of Dan: future business billionaire, supporting his aging parents in a manner to which they could easily become accustomed. He picked an easy language to learn, Mandarin. I liked the sound of "international emerging-markets business magnate." After his second year, he worked for a summer in Fuzhou, China, where his cousin Meredith's first husband Greg was an executive at McDonald's.

Then we got the call. Dan informed us that he was leaving college for a year to work in China, but he had no job yet. Who did he think he was, Bill Gates, Harvard dropout? Fern and I were petrified about his seemingly half-baked plans, but we went along after we made him promise that he would get an official leave of absence from Columbia and would return in a year to finish school. He kept his promise, first working for the American Chamber of Commerce in Shanghai and then for a local marketing firm that showed American products in neighborhood Chinese food markets. Doing this took some guts and initiative, a fact not lost on McKinsey and Company (neither was his being Phi Beta Kappa and summa cum laude), where he went to work in its Manhattan office for his first job after graduation.

We visited Dan during the year he was in China while we were on a tour sponsored by the University of Pennsylvania Alumni Association, which included several days in Shanghai. We introduced him to our tour buddies, and serving as the interpreter, he introduced us to his Chinese friends and showed us around. Dan lived in a regular working-class neighborhood, where a white face was an oddity, eliciting stares and smiles. We felt pretty proud of Dan.

Fern is a natural snoop. In another life, she would have made an excellent detective. While the kids were away, anything of interest in their rooms would be found and carefully examined. One day, I was peacefully reading a newspaper in the living room when I saw Fern at the top of the stairs, holding what looked like a letter and shrieking "Jeff, what's this? What does this mean?"

I took the letter from her. It was a letter to Dan from a female classmate, a friend who was away on a leave of absence. It was chatty, mostly tidbits about mutual friends. Toward the end was an almost offhand comment: "I'm so proud of you for COMING OUT" (my capitals).

I couldn't believe it. I'm a psychiatrist, Fern and I raised the kid, and we hadn't had the slightest suspicion that our son was gay. He wasn't effeminate and didn't play with dolls. It was true that he dated almost not at all in prep school, but I was like that too: studies came first. And he had a hot date for the senior prom. As far as we could tell, he had a number of girlfriends at Columbia. We met one, and she was bright and adorable. I even got a call from her father when Dan broke up with her, begging me to intervene because his little girl's heart was broken. In other words, we were clueless.

Fern understood what that letter clearly meant, and when I confirmed it, I was upset, and she was devastated. For me it meant changing my expectations of having a smart, probably Jewish daughter-in-law and brilliant grandkids too—I really wasn't sure what. For Fern it was much more earth-shattering, and for years she couldn't talk about it much with me or at all with anybody else.

A week or two later, Dan came home for a visit. I said, "Dan, we need to talk."

Dan looked pale.

"Is there something you need to tell us?"

"Like what?"

"Like that you're gay, that's what."

Then we showed him the letter.

"Where did you get that?"

"In the bottom of your desk," Fern said.

"You're not supposed to go through my things."

I replied, "If it's here, it's ours!" Then I lost it. "When were you gonna tell us? When you got AIDS?"

This was during the AIDS crisis, when many young, gay men were dying of acquired immune deficiency syndrome, and my fear for Dan made me harsh.

We went through the usual "We accept you and we love you," but of course it changed our sense of Dan and maybe of ourselves. Over the years we met many of the men Dan dated, and they seemed like terrific people.

Years later while in med school Dan met Jorge, and it was obviously very serious. Jorge was from Mexico, living in Manhattan and working at a high-end hotel. Their backgrounds were so different; he was Catholic and Latino, but he was a bright, sweet, good-looking guy, and the two had strong feelings for each other. It seemed that they planned to be together for good. My mother, Dan's Nana, didn't quite know what to make of it, which wasn't surprising given her generation and naturally conservative temperament. Her only eventual comment was "Jorge Portillo? Why not George Pearlstein?"

Eventually, Fern and I agreed that Dan should come out to the family at one of our annual Thanksgiving get-togethers. Dan would bring Jorge to the house to meet Jessica, Uncle Rick, Nana, and all my cousins and their kids.

Thanksgiving morning, Rick and I were shopping for some extras for the table, and I said, "Rick, there's something we need to talk about."

Rick gets nervous easily and asked, in his booming voice, "What? Is somebody sick? Is Jessica pregnant? Are you getting a divorce?"

"No, nothing like that. Dan's gay, and his boyfriend's a Mexican bellhop."

Rick visibly relaxed. "Is that why we're shopping? So you can blow shit in my ear?"

I repeated myself.

"Oy vey" was the best Rick could come up with.

The dinner actually went quite well. My cousins and the rest of the family couldn't have been friendlier. Mother didn't say much.

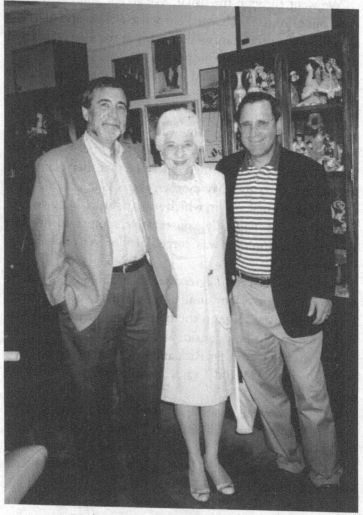

Mother and "Boys"—Thanksgiving in Danvers

Jessica in College and Weddings

Jess started at Northeastern University, a large city university in Boston. Initially she loved the school and made many friends there and enrolled in the physical therapy program. Unfortunately, she and physics didn't get along so well, so she changed to Spanish language and literature. She changed schools too, transferring to Brandeis, which she was convinced that Nana and I preferred.

I preferred that Jess be reasonably happy wherever she was and whatever she studied. There was a fair amount of drama and mood swings associated with all the changes, but she graduated from Brandeis ready to teach and travel.

As a kid, Jess never much liked to travel and preferred to go to camp in the summer. I took Dan to New York City and Washington, DC, one summer and to the US West the next, and Jessica stayed home. Somehow, Jessica decided to make up for lost time traveling all over the world teaching English as a second language—and probably getting into mishaps I'd sooner not know about. In Brazil she met her beloved, a med student named Bruno Schmitz.

Jess was absolutely convinced that Bruno was "the one," so of course Fern and I went down to Rio to meet him. He was a sweet, funny guy with a nice dad who was a professor of computer science at the Federal University in Rio, where Bruno was a med student.

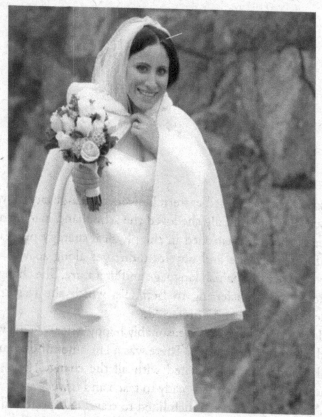

Beautiful Bride

Bruno's mom, whom we never met, was an ob-gyn in Rio. Apparently, Jessica was interfering with her plans to keep Bruno in Rio to open a medical lab, as Bruno was interested in pathology. Sparks flew between them, and at one point, objecting to our daughter's ideas about her beloved Bruno, his mom threw a heavy pot at Jessica.

Jess and Bruno's plan was for Bruno to come to the United States; they would live together while he prepared for licensure exams. They asked if I could help him get some kind of med student clerkship here.

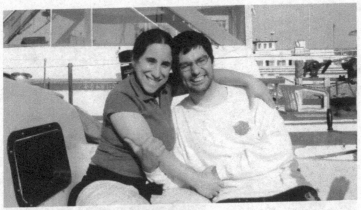

Jessica and Beloved

I had no direct connections, but I was part of a large consortium of hospitals affiliated with the Harvard Medical School. I cold-called two pathology departments, and amazingly, the pathology department at Brigham and Women's Hospital showed interest in Bruno. With Jess's help, Bruno filled out his application and got his clerkship.

After Bruno graduated from med school, he came here and lived with Jess. While she taught school, he prepared for his US board exams. Amazingly, he passed them all and wound up getting a residency at the University of Minnesota. At some point in this process Jess and Bruno eloped and got married in Las Vegas, and we had a party for them in Danvers.

I wondered if they were interested in a real Jewish wedding. I think Jess knew that I wanted to marry off my only daughter with a little style. We knew that this could be a major project, and I didn't want to push it too much, but Jess said okay, and of course Bruno went along. I was the only dad in the bridal gown store, which was odd but fun. Jess chose a simple but pretty gown. She was never more gorgeous.

The wedding was in Gloucester at a place called The Tavern, overlooking Gloucester Harbor. The food and music were

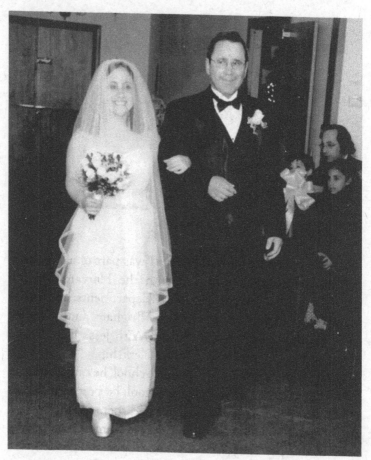

Proud Moment

great. They were married by a lady who was a lawyer turned Reformed cantor. Walking my only daughter down the aisle to "Sunrise, Sunset" was for me one of life's thrilling moments, as was celebrating with all our friends and family.

Two years later, Dan married Jorge. In many ways it was a traditional Jewish wedding, though clearly many of the guests had no idea what to expect. Fern and I walked Dan, garbed in a shroud over his suit, down the aisle. Jorge's mom,

Antonia, did the same with him. I'd never seen this, though Dan informed us that it was part of Jewish wedding tradition. Apparently Orthodox Jewish men get married in the same shroud in which they are buried. To me the symbolism is macabre, but according to the Talmud, it is intended as a poignant reminder that life is temporary and that it should be pursued in a meaningful, faithful way.

Okay, so it was a little weird walking Dan down the aisle to marry another man, but the wedding was a joyful one, with dancing and celebrating with our family and friends, only slightly marred by the fact that my mother, Dan's Nana, did not attend, pleading that she was too old and frail. Her frailty didn't prevent her from showing up for Dan's med school graduation just before that, though, a ceremony clearly more to her liking. I don't think Dan ever quite forgave her for not being there. And I had never seen Jess more beautiful with the exception of her own wedding.

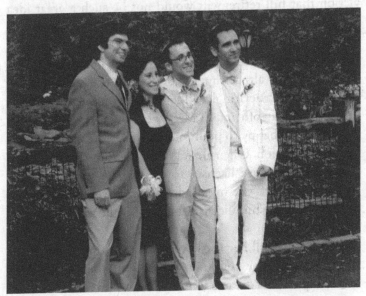

Dan and Ariel's NYC Wedding

Florida and Grandkiddies

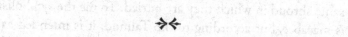

THE NEW ENGLAND WINTERS weren't getting any warmer despite the dire predictions of "warming" enthusiasts. As our children went on their paths with their spouses, we skied at Sunday River less. Eventually we rented it out, and finally, after owning it for about twenty years, we sold it. We still liked the idea of a vacation home of our own. My parents enjoyed being snowbirds in Florida for many years, and this appealed to both Fern and me. We anticipated that at some point we would retire to Florida too. Fern had the conviction that full retirement would not be such a great idea for me (for her, however, seven-day-per-week retirement to tennis seemed about right), so she insisted that I obtain a Florida medical license before we bought a home in Florida. This used to be almost impossible, but in the early 2000s it was merely excruciatingly difficult. I had a telephone relationship with an officious Tallahassee bureaucrat for about a year. She was happy to point out all the errors and do-overs in my application. One rule was that for some reason, I had to have three active licenses to qualify for one in Florida, so I had to reactivate my original Pennsylvania license and my New Hampshire licenses before I could even begin the Florida process.

I wanted to tell her to shove the application through the phone and up her you-know-where, but that would have ended my Florida dreams forever.

After a year, I got the Florida license and again deactivated the ones for Pennsylvania and New Hampshire. Now we were ready to shop for our Florida home.

We looked for two years, first up and down Florida's eastern coast, which we concluded was simply too crowded. We looked on the western coast from Manatee County down to Naples. I got an offer to work in a Naples practice, but we decided at that point that Florida was for vacations only. We eventually found a small new development called the Venetian Golf and River Club in Venice, a town in Sarasota County half an hour south of the city of Sarasota. The club had a beautiful golf course, six tennis courts, and, as the realtor, put it "a country-club lifestyle," which appealed to me. We bought a small house (fifteen hundred square feet) and vacationed there on weekends or for weeks at a time, sometimes with family or friends but mostly just Fern and me. It was then a community of mostly younger retirees from the Northeast, the Midwest, Canada, England, and Germany, but there was also a substantial minority of young families, with daily visits to the gate by our local school bus. Everyone was new to Florida and eager to meet people. It wasn't hard to make friends.

We spent our vacation weeks enjoying Venice and Sarasota eateries and theater, tennis (which I liked more than I thought I would) for me, golf (which I grew to cordially dislike but still duff at it with friends), and duplicate bridge, which I'm fair at but really enjoy. Mother advised me never to give it up (she played to age one hundred), because if I'm too old or frail for golf or tennis, bridge will be a good friend. I haven't reached that point yet, but it was good advice.

After five years we were ready. We were still not too old to enjoy all the amenities of Florida. I decided to close my practice and look for a larger home in the same development. Giving up the business of medicine was no sacrifice, but saying goodbye to my patients, some of whom I had treated for decades, was sad and painful on both sides.

I received a lot of gratitude and loving farewells. I expected more anger but experienced almost none, getting well wishes instead. I don't remember feeling guilty, but I was sadder than I anticipated. One reason it went smoothly is that I gave many months of advance notice, giving my patients the opportunity to find other doctors and work through their feelings about the separation. If it's possible I recommend this to any physician with patients of long standing, particularly psychiatrists.

Our plan was to be snowbirds, living half the year in Florida and half in Massachusetts. I would do locum tenens, which are temporary jobs in psychiatry that were readily available but were not as professionally satisfying as following your own patients. I did exactly one just after I closed my practice, a six-week stint on a very busy community hospital inpatient unit in Melrose, Massachusetts. It was intense and exhausting. I felt like an intern. I did a good job (the boss wanted me to stay longer), but as far as I was concerned, I had nothing to prove and was only interested in outpatient clinic practice.

Then I received a job offer from a community mental health center called Coastal Behavioral Healthcare, located near our new home in Florida. I asked for a maximum of three days a week and a minimum of two. The center offered me three. (I think I could have gotten eight.) No more billing, no more business worries; I could concentrate on just taking care of patients. But it would require living full-time in Florida. We decided to give it a try. We sold our house in Danvers and rented a nearby condo for a year. If the year worked out, fine. If not, we'd find another place in Massachusetts.

We found that we liked Florida even in the summer. It was hot but quiet, with rain and afternoon breezes off the Gulf of Mexico. The logistics and planning (selling our Danvers house, selling Sunday River, selling our small house in Florida, buying a larger house, moving from a house to an apartment, going to work in Florida) was stressful and complicated, and at one point we owned three properties (the Hoffmans of Danvers, Venice, and Newry, you know), but thanks to the fact that Fern was a superb detail woman, we got it done in stages over time.

Initially I started working with Coastal Behavioral Health-care at three different offices, in Venice, Sarasota, and Arcadia, a quirky little town fifty miles inland.

On my first day in Venice the clinic decided to "go easy," scheduling just a few patients. The first turned out to be a fifty-year-old woman who was in raging manic euphoria and was in urgent need of hospitalization. She of course didn't see it that way. She was enjoying life far too much and planned to leave the clinic for a jog on the local highway. So, we had to watch her and engage her for hours, waiting out the unbearably slow response of the local police and the ambulance, which to her loud disagreement transferred her to the psychiatric unit in Sarasota.

Arcadia was hard to pigeonhole: part Deep Dixie and part cowboy town (and participant in the national rodeo circuit), agricultural town, Mexican village, and home of cutesy antique boutiques. The patient mix was unusual, even by mental health clinic standards. One of my first was a young woman in her thirties I'll call "Tattoo Lady," all of whose visible skin (and there was a lot) was covered by tattoos. She presented very sad and weepy and was complaining of depression.

When I asked Tattoo Lady why she was depressed, she told me that she had just lost her baby girl, age three months. I nodded and asked her to tell me more, and she explained that she was nursing her baby when she fell asleep, and when she awoke, the baby was dead at her breast. It was horrible and bizarre beyond imagining, and I inadequately expressed my condolences.

Then Tattoo Lady began undoing her blouse. I panicked for a second, thinking of my Cindy experience many years before, but quickly realized that this biker chick was very unlikely to be looking to this old psychiatrist for that kind of consolation.

Tattoo Lady beckoned me to come closer to her now exposed left breast, and there was tattooed "Sweet Suzi, born [date], died [date]."

Frequently, Coastal Behavioral Healthcare patients have unending needs: financial, legal, drug- and alcohol abuse–related, chaotic dysfunctional families, and poor medical care.

Unlike in private practice, where the doctor with his or her therapist can meet the patients' mental health needs, often in collaboration with family or primary care physician, at Coastal Behavioral Healthcare, nurses, social workers, case planners, and inpatient psychiatric staff have to work as a team to help coordinate their many needs. Many have lives that go from crisis to crisis.

All of this is in addition to serious chronic mental illness and often inadequately treated medical illness. I loved that job.

Dan and Jorge, who took the name Ariel, moved from place to place following Dan's career. After his internship on Long Island they lived in a suburb of Detroit, Huntington Woods, while Dan did his dermatology residency at Henry Ford Hospital in Detroit.

It was there that Dan and Ariel adopted our grandchildren, four of them. Michael, the first but not the oldest, was two years old. He was a gorgeous, cherubic-looking, blond, blue-eyed boy, somewhat small in stature. Michael is one who listens to the beat of his own drummer—and stubbornly so. He is smart and articulate and can be utterly charming, but his priority is sometimes the whim of the moment, much to the consternation of his parents and teachers. Unfortunately, Michael developed a couple of serious medical issues, juvenile rheumatoid arthritis and juvenile diabetes, the former well controlled, the latter not so well because he loves sweets. I hope he develops a little restraint on this as he gets older. I think Michael could make a great defense lawyer when he gets around to concentrating in school.

Shiloh (pronounced Shilah) was adopted at age three and is six months older than Michael. While the others had been in foster care when they were adopted, Shiloh knew her mom, her grandmother, and her siblings and was wisely carefully transitioned away from her family of origin. She still has memories of them and has been encouraged to talk about them.

Shiloh is beautiful and also blond. She is exquisitely sensitive to the feelings of others and eager to please. She has a fierce sense of what's right and what isn't. Once on a playground, she saw a child pushing her younger African American brother and ran to his defense, yelling "You leave my brother alone!" The kid replied, "He can't be your brother." Shiloh screamed back, "Haven't you ever heard of adoption?"

Shiloh is probably the most naturally loving child I've ever known. She also has raging ADHD. At the end of the day, she can be all over the place. She always tries her best in her schoolwork, not so much out of innate interest as from a desire to please her parents and teachers. She is a very good athlete and loves basketball and skiing.

The younger two children, Boaz and Sharona, were adopted together. They are African American and are biological brother and sister. Boaz was two years old and Sharona one year old when they were adopted, and they'd both been in foster care from birth.

Boaz is outgoing, extremely affable, and impossible not to like. He is the most gifted athletically. I imagine that he will be a successful salesman or public relations guy some day.

Little Sharona is the shiest of the four, and it takes a while for her to trust you. She is adorable and remarkably conscientious and has a talent and patience for detail that eludes the

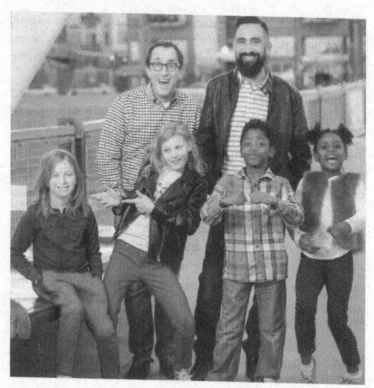

Dan, Ariel, and Family

other children. She is also gifted athletically, and I predict that she will excel academically.

Dan and Ariel have raised their children to be bilingual, and I'm told that they speak Spanish like little Mexicans. Their parents send them to Jewish camps in Mexico. Lucky kids!

Dan and Ariel keep an observant Jewish household, including Shabbat, the holidays, and kashrut. They send the children to Jewish day school. I see pros and cons but try to keep my nose out of their business when it comes to religion. Their kids' education and lifestyle are consistent with their parents' values and practices, and their children accept a Jewish life as natural to them.

Jess and Bruno moved around a lot too. After his residency at the University of Minnesota (where Jess got a master's degree in adult education), they moved to Jacksonville for a year, where Bruno did a fellowship in cytology, the pathology of individual cells and how to make diagnoses by looking at them.

Bruno's passion, apart from Jessica and his work, has always been airplanes, and he became a small-plane pilot. I think that his true desire would have been to become a US Navy jet fighter pilot. He did get the navy part and became a medical officer in the US Navy as a pathologist. Bruno was first stationed at Newport, Virginia, and then transferred to Bethesda, where Lieutenant Commander Bruno is on staff at Walter Reed. Meanwhile, Jess teaches English as a second language and adult high school classes at a local junior college. Her students love her wherever she is. It turns out that she's a born teacher.

Jess and Bruno always kept their family plans close to the vest. As far as we knew, our grandchild from them would be our granddoggie Kinko, a good-natured Sheltie.

In the late spring of 2014, I got the call. "Guess what, Dad. I'm pregnant." Jess was thirty-four, and this was unexpected. The pregnancy went fairly well, but at the end she developed preeclampsia and needed a C-section, and out came little Mario, a small but healthy boy who is the latest little light of our lives.

Jess and Bruno are great people, but easygoing is not an adjective that applies to either of them. So, it is hard to figure out how Mario got to be the placid child he is. He is also sweet-natured and naturally sociable toward everyone. He smiles easily and often, and at the nursery they fight over who gets to take care of him. I predict that he will turn out to be very smart and a lover (girls of all ages are already drawn to him). Since his father, uncle, and two of his grandparents are physicians, he has a natural pedigree (Penn Med, class of

2041?). His mother, two of his grandparents, and his great-grandma were teachers (one a college professor), so he has pedigrees in that direction too.

Bruno and Jess dote on each other and adore Mario. Their household can be a tad disorganized, but they are loving parents and will encourage Mario and get the best from him. Wait and see!

My dad died in 1995 of lung cancer at the age of eighty-three. He had smoked when he was young, but I never saw it. He led an active life almost to the end and was an avid racquetball player until he was about eighty. Before he died, my parents got to travel all over the world with their friends, and their memories are contained in many photo albums of their trips.

By today's standards, Dad was a violent father with a bad temper who hit easily and often, and I was afraid of him. I understand that in the early years he was under a great deal of pressure in a business he hated (the deli) but stayed in to please his own parents. I know that he had significant post-traumatic stress disorder from his combat in World War II, of which I was completely unaware as a child. I think that he was considered somewhat over the top with respect to his temper, even in those days. When my parents argued about it, my mother would say things like "You know, your friends call you Hitler behind your back."

My brother Rick, who had the bedroom adjacent to theirs on the third floor when he was a small child, often heard our father's nightmare screams of "Andy, Andy! Watch out!" Many years later, Rick told me about this. Andy was Dad's buddy in combat and was in the foxhole next to his when Andy got his head blown off.

Rick became a lawyer and settled in Tulsa, where he maintains his law practice. He's a brilliant guy with a photographic memory. He's also a sports nut, and we get together a couple of times a year to go to ball games. He never married, so Fern and I, our kids, and the grandkids are his family too, and we try to get together as much as we can.

Dad was a wonderful grandfather and could not do enough for Dan and Jessica. On vacations in Philadelphia or Florida, Mom and Dad would watch the kids for days while Fern and I took many a minivacation. Harry and Doris, Fern's parents, did the same for us in Philadelphia. My dad was also an amazing financial planner and, by making careful investments with their pension funds, supported Mother well for the twenty-one years she lived as a widow.

Mother and Dad had just bought a new home in Boynton Beach, Florida, where they planned to live full-time for the rest of their days. Unfortunately, Dad only lived another year. Mother continued to live at Palm Isles, a resort-like retirement community, where she enjoyed many friends as well as her passionate hobby, bridge.

There Mother remained for fifteen relatively happy years until at age ninety-five she concluded that taking care of her

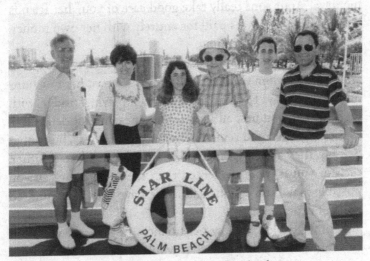

Visit with Mother and Dad—Florida

own place was getting to be "too much." Mother was a very practical woman with little sentimentality or illusions about her capabilities.

In fact, Mother was entering the early stages of dementia.

Rick, Fern, and I all agreed that we would all be better off if Mother lived close to us, so we did a diligent search of local places that might be suitable. Filling the bill was Kobernick House, a middle-class kosher Jewish independent-living facility that had access to an assisted-living facility, a memory unit, and a rehab/nursing facility. The independent-living units included studios, one bedrooms, two bedrooms, and a few large ultraluxury two bedrooms, the only units with their own washer and dryer.

Mom moved into one of the ultraluxury two bedrooms, and I suppose social status there had something to do with the size of your unit. Her friends there—and she made many—often asked, "What do you need a place that big for?" She would give vague answers such as "My sons think it's best."

Mom loved the envy, I'm sure, and when she got such comments as "Your sons really take good care of you," her friends had no idea that it was paid for entirely with her own money, thanks to my dad's planning.

Despite her memory gradually failing as well as her vision and hearing, Mom managed to play bridge past her one hundredth birthday. I once witnessed her playing bridge with three of her buddies, all in their nineties and all demented. None of them could remember whose deal it was, but unbelievably, they all played incredibly well. I asked her, "Mother, each of you is more demented than the next. How can you possibly play bridge?" She said, "We have over two hundred years of experience."

Mother couldn't follow her finances in the later years but constantly worried about what would happen if she ran out of money. Rick and I assured her that we had a backup plan.

We had a lovely cardboard box and a nice spot picked out for her under a bridge in Venice. I promised to visit her every few days, rain or shine. I know that reassured her.

We had a sweet hundredth birthday party for Mom at the Sarasota Ritz, attended by her good friend Liz, Rick, Fern, me, Dan, Jessica, grandsons-in-law Ariel and Bruno, her nephews David and Howard along with Howard's wife Naomi, and David's girlfriend, Pat. Jessica gave Mom a sash that said "Birthday Girl 100 Years Old." Mother shed quite a few happy tears.

The dinner and speeches were in a private dining area, and as Mother walked out of the dining room in her sash, she got a standing ovation from the bar customers. Mother waved at them like a Hollywood diva.

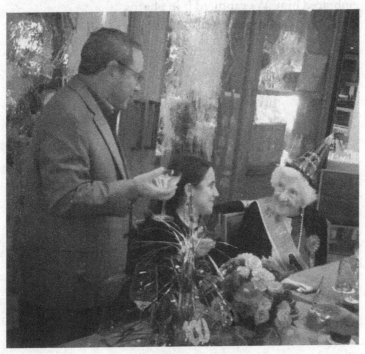

Nana's 100th Birthday

Over the next year and a half Mother faded quickly and had a number of hospitalizations for infectious illnesses. By then she required 24/7 private-duty nursing to stay in her apartment at Kobernick, and she finally reached the point that she wasn't getting any further benefit from living there. Rick and I decided that the next time she was hospitalized and transferred to the Kobernick rehab, she would remain in the nursing facility. Unfortunately, we correctly predicted that soon she wouldn't remember that she once lived elsewhere. I tried to visit Mother regularly, and Rick remained in touch by phone, visiting when he could.

In late August 2016, Jess and Bruno came to visit with little Mario, then seven months old. Mario was placed in the bed to meet his great-grandma. They smiled at each other, and she embraced him. We captured it in photos.

Mother died about a week later.

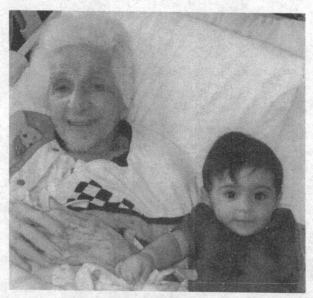

Mother with Great-Grandson Mario

Conclusion

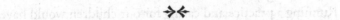

I WAS THE FIRST SON of working-class Jewish parents who themselves were children of the Great Depression. They grew up in a world where anti-Semitism was more blatant and economic opportunity for Jews seemed limited. They were fearful for me and my brother, afraid that without constant prodding we would have miserable lives.

Mother mostly called the shots, relying on advice from friends and family on matters educational, secular, religious, musical, and athletic, and Dad went along.

My parents were absolutely right in the conviction that my only certain future lay in my ability to do well in school and that if I weren't pushed for top grades I could easily slack off. They had a good point. Like the tiger parents of today, providing a "happy childhood" was pretty irrelevant.

Do I regret going to med school? Absolutely not. Would I have wound up there without the push? Doubtful.

I wound up in a specialty that worked for me. It required a certain empathy and patience, for which I had a knack. In psychiatry, diagnosis and treatment plan are the easy part. Gaining the trust of suffering individuals who may think and act uniquely because of the way their minds operate and then creating a therapeutic alliance is the true challenge in my field. You have to imagine thinking like a paranoid, a borderline personality, or a depressed, hopeless person before you can help patients help themselves.

Advances in neuroscience, genetics, and psychopharmacology, not to mention general medical advances, are sure to make our field continuously interesting, and it deserves to attract the brightest students.

Running a practice and caring for our children would have been impossible without Fern. She has been an incredible helpmate, steady, reliable, and totally caring. She has had the tougher job.

I can't imagine how empty life would feel for me without our children, Dan and Jessica. I'm not saying that they haven't been total pains in the ass at times, but they have somehow become responsible and decent adults and now have their own families. Astonishingly, they still look to Mom and Dad for advice sometimes.

Fern and I were much less assertive about our kids' choices than our parents were, at least partly because we did not have the economic insecurities of our parents. My parents were deathly afraid of the possibility that we would have the financial problems they'd had, so they made damn sure that we entered professions that would prevent that. We didn't worry so much about our kids and encouraged them to find their own way.

I've done two kinds of practices in my career, the first more or less middle class, with patients ranging from the very poor to very wealthy. For the last several years I've served in a different setting, taking care of mostly poor people in a clinic.

They are beset by constant financial problems, family problems, substance abuse, legal worries, and poor or inadequate medical care, all in addition to chronic, serious mental health problems such as schizophrenia, severe bipolar disorder, ADHD, depression, and post-traumatic stress disorder, which have been my primary responsibility to treat. Incredible levels of stress often constitute their daily lives. I've needed the help of social workers, case managers, therapists, and psychiatric nurses, all contributing their skills to help me to do what I do.

Yet these patients have seemed to me particularly grateful for my efforts, and sometimes my listening, in combination with my psychiatric cocktails, seems to actually make a difference for the better in the quality of their lives.

I'm very lucky for that.

Occasional Poems

How Bruno and Jessica Got Hitched

Now Jess our dear daughter will gather no rust
She suffers a case of severe wanderlust
She's wandered the globe a free spirit at will
And last year in Rio to teach in Brazil
From emails adventures told happy and sad
The phone just for big news (the good or the bad)
The phone rings, its Jess, "I'm just fine, you the same?
My new boyfriend's a med student, Bruno's his name
This guy is the best: he's the one I adore."
(But haven't we heard that a few times before?)
"Oh Mom oh Dad how happy I feel"
So we flew down to Rio to get them a meal
And while we were there it was also our mission
To settle the question of Bruno's ambition
He answered "To sail and to fly and oh yes
To be a Path Resident in the US."
He was smart and was funny but more to the point
The glow in their eyes really lit up the joint
By the time we had finished our first Rio dinner
We knew that for sure Jess had picked her a winner
So Jessie and Bruno to Boston they dash
For Jessie to teach and to make them some cash

For Bruno a clerkship at old Harvard Med
And to study for med boards (if he don't pass he's dead)
But time it runs short on prolonged visa stays
In Canada, they are told there are ways
So that if they go there with no more delays
The Brazilian Consulate adds ninety days
But there at the border a grim shock awaits
When Jessie and Bruno try leaving the States
The guard says to Bruno "You can cross if you will
If you try to return your butt's back to Brazil"
"Oh Jessica dear, I don't mean to be rude
But it sure looks as though we have really got screwed"
With a gleam in her eye she asks "Oh tell me Bru,
Do you love me as much as is my love is for you?"
"Jess you know that I do, that we're soul mates, a team"
"Then here's my idea for fulfilling our dream"
So a few nights later my telephone rings
Jess talking in circles 'bout green cards and things
"Please get to the point, Jess, before I stroke out"
"Well this is good news, Dad, no reason to pout
This green card perplexity left us so harried
So we flew to Las Vegas and got ourselves married
The lawyer assured us it was the best way
We were going to do it next year anyway
It wasn't impulsive, we thought it all through"
"Of course you did, Jess, just like you always do"
So I sighed, turned to Fern and asked "Please let me hear
Just what it is you think of Bruno, my dear?"
"Oh he's great" was her answer, "with hardly a flaw"
"You better think that, he's our new son-in-law"
Welcome family and friends, hope you're feeling well fed
Now lets raise a toast to our new newlyweds.

For Anne and Lou's Fiftieth

How do two people who're wed fifty years
prosper, continue to thrive?
How to stay married for fifty years?
remarkable just to survive.
Successful examples so rare to choose,
we're here to celebrate Anne's and Lou's!

Anne traveled from Gloucester, George Kline's younger
    daughter
Temple U. Oral Hygiene to start.
And the rumors still tell, While with Bob and Adele
she broke many a Dent student's heart.

And Lou was the pride of the Yankel and Merrill
so deeply devoted a son.
He stayed close to home, How far could he roam?
with the family business to run.

Now Lou with ladies exceedingly shy
so he hung with Bones, Mutzy, and Al.
And Al was a swinger as everyone knew
and women he always had more than a few.
So Lou's social approach was
"Al, make it for two."

One fateful night Anne met her quiet Lou
the intro by Sylvia Pett.
And she knew in an instant (well one month or two)
the dentists she soon would forget.

And Anne captured Lou with her New England chaahm,
all bashfulness banished, all fears.

With decisive intent Lou would ask for her hand
the marriage took place in five years.

The wedding occurred on a quiet Spring day
at the homestead of Bob and Adele.
Lou was a G.I., and the world was at war
awaiting him, battlefield hell.

The honeymoon brief and both happy and sad
uncertainty made passion burn.
Before it was through Lou left Anne with a prize
he'd share with her if he'd return.

With the winter storm mounting
9 months 4 days (who's counting?),
Anne with Minnie and Max on Pine Street.
Doovv and Howard would fight,
While Don shoveled all night,
then Jeff entered the world by his feet.

The hours were long, but the corned beef a treat
at Hoffman's Deli on 29th Street
The family worked from dawn to dark
and sometimes they'd stroll out to Fairmount Park.

But in four years things got to be really tricky
when arrived an adorable bundle named Ricky.
Then did family serenity hit the skids,
were we really the world's two most rotten kids?

As a big brother Jeffrey's devotion was swell
to see to it Ricky's existence was hell.
For teasing and torment Jeff learned every trick
recall the crib lesson in arithmetic?

Sundays with the boys they'd make family rounds
to visit Dzubas, Blocks, Basses, or Browns.
And Anne and Lou would chat the whole day
while Jeff and Rick and the other kids play.

Also Lou's cousins
he had quite a few.
The Factor clan meetings and
Spring picnics too.

And Anne in the summer, the kids to the shore
to A.C. or Gloucester the family would pour.
To Irving's apartment we'd fit ten or more
and Lou came some weekends, his folks watched the
    store.

To do the hard work they were perfectly glad
to provide opportunities they never had.
And as for advantages let me tell you
those kids had advantages up the wazoo.

Anne schlepped them to concerts and schlepped them
    to swimming,
to Gratz, tennis and music that's just a beginning.
And if they'd complain to her or if they'd whine
she'd say you'll appreciate all in good time

You think all that effort just went down the drain
have you ever heard Jeffrey play "Lady of Spain"?

With Anne teaching school for some income expansion
the Hoffmans had finally got out of "The Mansion."
So upwardly mobile the family strode
to a leafy treed street that was called Lynnewood Road,

And scrimping and saving and guiding and planning
potential careers for their sons they were scanning.
Whatever they wanted, Anne couldn't be coyer
as long as it was either doctor or lawyer.

Forsaking all kinds of material joys
to collegiately educate two Jewish boys
Some screaming some nagging much caring and then
to hopefully give the world two decent men.

Their sons moving on to form lives of their own
the first time for Anne and Lou really alone.
And if you think this was a matter for grief
then you've never raised kids, 'twas a sigh of relief.

Approaching the upcoming years with much zest
from travel and racquetball, concerts no rest.
With family bar mitzvahs and bridge games to play
and a new place called home that was named Baker's Bay.

"Oh, hi folks, It's Jeff, And I'm going to marry
my beautiful Fern, child of Doris and Harry
A daughter-in-law and two great muchetunem
A nice Jewish girl with a cute shainem punem
So Mother, please take your head out of the oven."

"Just one favor son from your dad and your mother
can you please talk the same sense as yours to your
    brother."

But Rick would have none of this settling down
and wandered out west down to old Tulsa town
"Please give us a call Rick, Jeff helps with our pills"
"Don't worry, I'll gladly strike Jeff from your wills"

In '78, '80 two joys come anew
the arrivals of Daniel and Jessica too.
They'll always be Mother and Dad it is true
for Mom "call me Nana," and Dad "Grandpa Lou."

The family visits not frequent and yet
the happiest moments that Anne and Lou get.
And how can I speak for all days that they live?
I know what they get 'cause I know what they give.

The give time and attention and humor and the sharing
of kindness and interest, unconditional caring.
The feelings created will warm the insides
of their kids and grandkids for the rest of our lives.

And sadly reminded we make an admission
pain and grief are a part of the human condition.
And like all of you Anne and Lou's had their share
of sadness and loss and of burdens to bear.

Does this mean that 50's an end well No Way!
there's a lot of good years and good life from today.
We wish them good weather good friends and all
    smiles
enjoying their beautiful home in Palm Isles.

So how does a marriage that lasts 50 years prosper,
    continue to thrive?
Companionship partnership family and friends
that keeps the glow bright and alive.

With Love From
Rick, Jeff, Fern
Dan, and Jessica

The Last Time I Went Fishing with Roger

The time I went fishing with Roger, he was closer to
    four than five-Oh
And if memory serves me correctly, 'twas at least two
or three boats ago

The day was a warm one in summer
the ocean was smooth as you please
The temp was a comfortable seventy-five
with barely a hint of a breeze

As we gingerly boarded the vessel
which he showed me around with great pride
It was clean it was new; he the Chief, I the crew
'twas a glorious day for a ride

So I put my week's work far behind me
all the crazies me stressed to the max
I had only one plan, one intent, I began
to settle me down and relax.

As we made our way out past the harbor
and far out upon open seas
We downed one or two of Rog's favorite brew
while feeling completely at ease.

When suddenly nudged from my reverie,
I noted the motor subside.
Rog says, "Put down your beer, we drop anchor right here,"
so we tossed it over the side.

"Now Jeffrey, you know why we're out here,
to catch many a fish before night

And when out here with me, as soon you will see,
I'll show you how fishing's done right."

Now perhaps I was slightly offended
Did he think my life spent on the shore?
Did he know of my salt fishing history past
(Well at least two or three times before)

And besides what the heck was the big deal
as the densest of dummies could state
Why all that it took, put the clam on the hook,
drop the line in the water and wait.

Now Rog glanced at me with forbearance
though I felt like I'd brains of an ox
And "Jeffrey," he said, "This is nothing to dread
let me show you my new tackle box."

As I looked deep inside this collection
of hooks, bobs, and lures by the slew,
Well I just never dreamed deep sea fishing involved
so many choices for you.

"Now Jeff," old Roger assured me,
"this is simply a novice's gear.
And I don't want to gloat, but in front of this boat
is the latest in SONAR this year."

Now I found this a little confusing;
of the fine points of tackle unsure.
He explained on and on, my attention span gone,
I said, "Rog, why don't you pick the lure?"

Well next came the matter of casting the rod,
for me this was really old hat
Snap the reel with a twist, then a flick of the wrist
now what could be simpler than that?

And I reached back the rod and released it,
over the side with a whip.
But Rog looked with dismay, "Jeff, it's the wrong way.
Now here, let me show you the grip."

And so it went all through the afternoon,
all fine points which Rog had to say,
of baiting and casting and playing the fish,
a most educational day.

But one thing that left me quite puzzled
this really did not make much sense.
After all the relaxing and fishing and learning,
Now why was I feeling so tense?

No matter; we all have our leisurely styles
lax or obsessional zest.
But we know whatever dear Roger pursues
will be done at perfectionist's best.

You may want to know at the end of the day
regarding the afternoon's take
By the evening so still; we put gas to the grill
and dined on a sizzling steak.

Happy Fiftieth Roger and many fun-filled years to
    follow!

                                    Jeff and Fern Hoffman

Printed in the USA
CPSIA information can be obtained
at www.ICGtesting.com
JSHW031714140824
68134JS00038B/3684

9 781635 765618